# Detoxification and HEALING

# Detoxification and HEALING

## THE KEY TO OPTIMAL HEALTH

SIDNEY MACDONALD BAKER, M.D.

*Foreword by Jeffrey S. Bland, Ph.D.*

KEATS PUBLISHING, INC.          *New Canaan, Connecticut*

Detoxification and Healing: The Key to Optimal Health

Copyright © 1997 by Sidney MacDonald Baker, M.D.

All Rights Reserved

No part of this book may be reproduced in any form without the written consent of the publisher.

Library of Congress Cataloging-in-Publication Data

Baker, Sidney M.
    Detoxification and healing / by Sidney Baker,
        p.   cm.
    Includes bibliographical references and index.
    ISBN 0-87983-709-8
        1. Metabolic detoxication.    2. Orthomolecular therapy.    I. Title.
    RM235.5.836   1997
    613—dc20                                                    98-46373
                                                                    CIP

Printed in the United States of America

Keats Publishing, Inc.
27 Pine Street (Box 876)
New Canaan, Connecticut 06840-0876

98  97  96     6  5  4  3  2  1

# Acknowledgments

WHILE WRITING THIS BOOK I have been like an anesthetized patient numbed by the ongoing urgency to write new pages and oblivious to many of the realities of my surroundings. An absent mind, interruptions, the loss of evenings by the fire and sunny days in the canoe make life difficult for the family of someone trying to write a book. Please join me in thanking my wife, Natalia, for not only putting up with all this but contributing her ideas and editorial skills.

Now that I am in the recovery room you can tell me if what was extracted from me in my operation was able to cure my need to communicate ideas that are not mine but come from various teachers, of whom my patients have been the best. The first, however, was Richard Mayo-Smith, my biology teacher at Phillips Exeter Academy, who rescued me from the illusion that science was all math and facts. He introduced me to the notion of ideas: that what we make of the facts depends on our ability to conceive of a framework in which to see the facts.

The late Linus Pauling based his perceptions about the molecular basis for treatment of illness on two very simple ideas: 1. Everyone is different and 2. Each individual's health benefits from having "the right molecules in the right amounts." His lectures in courses given for physicians at Stanford inspired me to follow medical paths that obey these two precepts, which Dr. Pauling called "orthomolecular medicine" (meaning the "right molecules medicine"). The medical profession's rejection of his notions made it professionally risky to identify oneself as a doctor with orthomolecular leanings. However, a growing number of health professionals are joining the many lay people who believe that before turning to medications we should attempt to adjust the normal body constituents to match needs for optimal functioning. I hope that a recognition of the orthomolecular implications of much of the current literature in nutritional medicine will lead to a renewed acceptance of orthomolecular medicine.

My friend, Leo Galland, M.D., and I worked together for several years a decade ago. Then and now Leo was a source of ideas and information that have been essential to the foundations of this book.

Another student of Dr. Pauling, Dr. Jeffrey Bland, has been the most influential teacher of physicians in the past two decades. Like many of my colleagues who set about to relearn biochemisty long after passing Part I Board Exams at the end of the second year of medical school, I owe him my ongoing thanks for his thoughtful and encyclopedic sifting of the current medical literature. I also owe special thanks to Dr. Jon Pangborn of Biognostic Laboratories, West Chicago, Illinois. Twenty years ago Jon set about to turn his knowledge of biochemistry into useful tools for gaining insight into individual biochemistry. Since then he has invested enormous amounts of time, energy and his impeccable integrity for the benefit of doctors and their patients who are looking for the biochemical basis of chronic health problems.

Other teachers and colleagues whose influence and ideas appear in this book are Drs. Karl Ernst Schaefer, Otto Wolff, Theron Randolph, Joe Beasley, Clyde Hawley, Phyllis Saifer, Larry Dickey, Frank Waickman, William Rea, Martin Lee, Stephen Barrie, John Rebello, James Braly, Orion Truss, Paul Cheney, Lloyd Saberski, William Crook, Leonard McEwen, Charles L. Remington and my friend Colin Furness whose friendship and advice have helped illuminate the path that made writing this book possible.

My most consistent teachers have been my patients. The lessons of a few of them are retold in this book. Hundreds of others have helped shape me as a physician as I developed the skills of explaining things that I have used in writing this book. The even more important skills of listening, listening again, and going over the story yet another time in the quest for clues to clinical puzzles are not so clearly evident in the chapters of this book in which I have chosen relatively simple cases. Becoming a good listener has been my principal aim as I have learned to respect the deep knowledge and intuition that my patients have about their bodies. What they lack is a scientific vocabulary, so that their initial efforts to explain their perceptions about their illness and its causes offend a scientific ear that has not been tuned to hear the signal through the noise.

My clinical assistants over the past 30 years have contributed their own listening skills to my own and helped create the time and space and atmosphere for listening in my office. They are Jayne Barese, RN, Gail Sherry, RN, Lisa Young, RMA, Veronica Brown, RMA, Dell Lamoureux, LPN, Maureen McDonnell, RN and Nancy Miller, RN.

My special thanks go to my brother, David E. Baker, whose enduring love and support have added to the strength needed to complete many of the tasks I have undertaken. To my daughters, Jennifer and Laura, I will always be grateful for their loyal love and forbearance during the time I have taken out to write.

I never sit for long at the keyboard without feeling the inspiration of my main model for writing, Louise Bates Ames, Ph.D., cofounder of the Gesell Institute and my friend and mentor since the time I worked with her there. The staccato of her typewriter was the music heard up and down the stairs of the old Victorian mansion on Prospect Street from 1950 until her recent death at age 88 in October 1966. No one in my life has provided for me a better model for candor, wit, persistence and value placed on the practical application of scientific insight.

Thanks to Drs. Louis Magnardli, John Anderson and Bill Kriski for their answers to my questions concerning toxic ticks.

Phyllis Herman has improved my manuscript with her keen eye and thoughtful suggestions. Karen Mahoney provided valuable research assistance.

# Contents

*Foreword by Jeffrey S. Bland, Ph.D.*      xi

*Preface*      xv

1. The Unity of the Immune System and the Central Nervous System      1

2. The Care and Feeding of the Permanent Cells: A Case of Infertility      10

3. Toxicity from Without: The Ambassador's Daughter      15

4. Toxic Hormones: A Boy with Breasts      23

5. Toxins from the Gut      28

6. Food as Toxin      39

7. You Are *Not* What You Eat      50

8. Fat Is Not Just to Hold Your Pants Up      54

9. DNA: The Family Jewels      73

10. Peptides from Foods: Molecular Masquerade      85

11. Dirty Smoke: Genetic Mistakes and Metabolic Abnormalities      93

12. Dietary Fiber and Hormone Regulation      104

13. The Many Faces of Gluten Intolerance      109

14. The Map: A Guide to Thoroughness in Approaching Health Problems      121

15. How Detoxification Works                         138
16. Rhythmic Harmony and Breathing                   162
17. Some Final Thoughts                              170
    *References*                                     181
    *Index*                                          191

# Foreword

In every discipline there are a few "master teachers," upon whose shoulders rests responsibility for the growth and evolution of the discipline, and for shaping its impact in the world. In the field of functional medicine and the practice of "good medicine," Sidney MacDonald Baker, M.D. is a master teacher. His new book, *Detoxification and Healing: The Key to Optimal Health,* might be called "A Great Doctor's Guide to the Practice of Good Medicine." Dr. Baker not only practices good medicine, but he knows how to communicate it to others, especially his patients. In this book he explains that illness is a complex phenomenon involving interplay among a person's belief system, environment and genetic structure, and the ability to defend him/herself against disorganizing forces. The body's defense is maintained by barriers including the skin, gastrointestinal mucosa, cellular membranes and the compartmentalization of organ systems that reserve certain functions in certain places in the body. When psychosocial or environmental factors, communicable organisms or the body's own expression of vitality bring about the breakdown of this organization of structure and function, the result is disease.

As a metaphor for facing the disorganizing factors that can cause disease, I recall Dr. Baker's discussion of his fear of roller coasters. Photographing a number of individuals as they rode over the top of a roller coaster, he found their responses to this disorganizing stimulus ranged from euphoria and bliss to the terror of impending doom. The same stimulus was met by widely differing responses. Dr. Baker believes this metaphor illustrates what happens in the disease process. We are all exposed to stimuli to which the body must respond—fast-paced lifestyle, environmental toxins, the foods we eat, communicable organisms, to name a few. Much like cresting the peak of the roller coaster ride, our bodies may respond with bliss and organized control, or with trauma and illness. The way one's body responds to these stimuli is in part related to the way he or she prepared for the ride up that first hill. Good nutrition, stress management, regular activity, and defending the body's protective barriers can make the ride more enjoyable and less risky. Having told his listeners of his fear of roller coasters, Dr. Baker concluded his talk by showing a picture of himself coming over the top of the ride. His arms were raised to the sky and he wore a blissful smile on his face. He had prepared himself well and found a way not only to survive but to enjoy the ride.

This metaphor is applicable to your reading of Dr. Baker's book. You will prepare yourself for the roller coaster ride of life by learning to mobilize organizational factors to improve and support your health rather than focusing on the gloom and doom of impending disease stimulus to which your body has no resilience.

You will be impressed by the way this master teacher weaves complex science into a program that is understandable, interesting, and applicable to your life. Dr. Baker explains, for example, the complex interaction between the external world and the internal world of gastrointestinal flora (bacteria). He points out that life and health are measured in part by the interplay of friendly, symbiotic bacteria that can help us and potentially health-damaging parasitic, toxic bacteria.

He explains that the relationships among gastrointestinal function, diet, environment and the living bacteria in our intestinal tract can support or alarm our immune system, with a resulting myriad of effects on the body. Over a period of time, if toxic exposure continues and the body responds with alarm reactions, the result is tissue destruction and the breakdown of barriers of defense of the body, and the disorganization we call illness.

It takes someone with Dr. Baker's skill to take sophisticated ideas out of the research laboratory and apply them responsibly to the needs of people who are ill, creating an accurate perception of the relative risks and benefits of these concepts. Dr. Baker has the ability to sift and screen information and reconnect it in a way that results in positive application by chronically ill patients who are looking for a path to restored health. Dr. Baker describes what he calls the "tack rules." If you are sitting on three tacks, he explains, you have to remove all three before you have significant reduction of discomfort. Pulling one or two tacks out and taking medication to relieve the pain caused by the third does not lead to the success one achieves by identifying all three precipitating factors and removing all three tacks.

By reading *Detoxification and Healing: The Key to Optimal Health,* you will find better ways of identifying the tacks that may be contributing to your particular discomfort and, better yet, learn ways to remove them all so that your body's positive, recuperative powers can be realized. Most of us possess recuperative powers and resilience in our health far greater than we ever expect, but because we have so many overlapping, precipitating factors that have not been identified, we never allow our bodies to achieve optimal function. Dr. Baker helps us identify the factors that contribute to reduced vitality and prepare ourselves to enjoy the vitality and bliss that can come from riding confidently on the roller coaster of life.

Enjoy the voyage of discovery with *Detoxification and Healing,* and recognize the art that comes from the master teacher's ability to make complex scientific information understandable and accessible for the maintenance and enhancement of health.

Jeffrey S. Bland, Ph.D.
CEO, HealthComm International, Inc.

# Preface

IT TAKES ABOUT 25 YEARS for a new idea to catch on in medicine. That is the time required for it to be tested in the crucible of science and become accepted as official policy. For example, there was sufficient information available in 1975[1] for a young woman to reasonably assume that taking a supplement of the B vitamin folic acid in pregnancy would prevent certain severe birth defects in her child. During the two decades it has taken for the folic acid connection to birth defects to be proven, thousands of babies have been born who might have been spared serious defects if their mothers had been able to make a personal choice based on their reading of the research instead of waiting for folic acid supplementation to become public policy. I am talking about ideas, not drugs, devices or procedures, although they have a similar time line from emergence to acceptance. This book will help you grasp current ideas and watch them catch on. You may want to accept these ideas as they apply to your personal health well before they have achieved the cachet of official acceptance. You may also want to consider many of the ideas in this book that will never be subjected to the rigorous and expensive processes needed to prove their validity.

*Cyberhealth:* I define cyberhealth as the application of the kind of thinking embodied in general systems theory to medicine. Cyberhealth has mostly to do with the approach one takes to understanding what has caused an event, such as a symptom or the collection of symptoms, signs and lab tests we call an illness. At present, medical thinking remains quite linear and simple. Doctors and patients alike are tempted by the idea that an illness has a single cause that can be treated with a single pill. General systems theory presents ideas about causality in which a web of interactions produce a result that is not as easy to blame on a single factor. Health is sustained by a state of balance among countless strands of a web of genetic, physiologic, psychological, developmental and environmental factors. When something goes wrong, it makes sense to pay attention to all aspects of this web that can be addressed with reasonable cost and risk. The occasional reference to cyberhealth in this book is a shorthand for the application of the principles of general systems theory to medicine.

There are two meanings of the word *systems*. When I became a doctor I learned about systems as a way of dividing the body and categorizing diseases that affect it. There are the cardiovascular, nervous, immune, reproductive, gastrointestinal, urinary, integumentary (skin), musculoskeletal, endocrine, reticuloendothelial and hematologic systems. In my medical training all my textbooks and all my courses were organized according to these divisions of the body. The same systems are the basis for classifying disease. When I graduated from medical school I was expected to pick a system and become a specialist. I could not decide on my favorite system. I did some training in obstetrics and completed my training in pediatrics to help me understand human development. I have remained a generalist and still stumble when the person in the next seat on an airplane asks me what kind of doctor I am. I never say that I am a specialist in cyberhealth.

I finished my specialty training in pediatrics in 1969 and, rather than taking a fellowship in heart, kidney or liver, I spent two years as the junior member in the new section of Medical Computer Science at Yale Medical School. Dean Fritz Redlich had conceived the idea of a computer section devoted not to number crunching but to finding ways to make computers useful in the day-to-day practice of medicine. My mentor was Dr. Shannon Brunjes, who began his academic career by specializing in the adrenal gland. His research entailed the use of computers. From Shannon I learned about systems theory in which the notion of system is quite different from the accepted medical way of dividing the body. Systems theory provides a unifying, as opposed to divisive, concept of how things work in nature as well as in computers. It allowed me to view biological systems as unified by the interaction of their many components and to make functional, as opposed to anatomical divisions, as I assessed balance within the whole system.

The medical concept of systems and disease leads a doctor toward a narrow path. The student doctor learns to take pride in a parsimonious approach to finding the one explanation for the patient's problem. The doctor gives the diagnosis, the name of the disease, as the explanation of the patient's problem and is comfortable saying that the disease is the cause of the symptoms. "Your sadness is being caused by depression," "Your high blood pressure is the result of hypertension," "Your cramps and diarrhea are being caused by colitis," "Your child can't pay attention because he has attention deficit disorder." Having made the diagnosis, the doctor may then apply the treatment that works best for that symptom: an antidepressant for depression, an antihypertensive for hypertension, a pill to suppress cramps and diarrhea, or Ritalin for the hyperactive child, a drug that would lead to the imprisonment of anyone found selling it near the playground.

Doctors who adhere to the emerging concepts of systems theory follow a broad path. Students of this approach take pride in a lavish approach that considers all the components of the patient's system that might be out of balance. The doctor makes a functional assessment with the understanding that the diagnosis is the name, not the cause, of the patient's symptoms. Having made the diagnosis, the doctor makes a functional assessment of the *individual* patient's balance and prescribes the supplementation of needed elements and the removal of toxic elements that interfere with balance. The broad path is less costly in the long run because it is faithful to the realities of the interrelationships in biological systems.

In 1959 I was a premed student just finished with nine months of traveling and studying Asian art history with my teacher Nelson Wu, when I went to work with Dr. Edgar Miller in Kathmandu, Nepal for three months before returning to my senior year at Yale. I had the privilege of being Dr. Miller's sidekick and assistant when he saw patients as part of his affiliation with Shanta Bhawan, a missionary hospital that, in the 1950s, represented the first presence of outsiders in the Kingdom of Nepal. Dr. Miller had retired at age 65 from his cardiology practice in Wilmington, Delaware and, with his wife, Elizabeth, a pediatrician, had joined the staff of what was then the only well-staffed, well-equipped medical facility in the valley of Kathmandu. In weekly clinics in outlying villages we saw patients who would line up at dawn to wait for Dr. Miller and his small team of Nepalese helpers and me. In spite of the dust, the crowded quarters provided on the second story of a village dwelling, the heat and the pressure to see every patient and return to Kathmandu the same day, Dr. Miller would turn to me after assessing each patient and ask, "Sidney, have we done everything we can for this patient?" I can hear the sound of his voice as I write these words and as I could all through my medical training when none of my other teachers ever posed such a question in such a way.

Dr. Miller's question takes on a different significance for a generalist and a systems analyst than it does for a specialist, a person focusing on one particular system. It is not just a question of the generalist concentrating on a large territory and the specialist on a restricted one. It is the kind of question that goes with systems theory as applied to medicine versus the present model in medicine that views the disease, not the individual as the target of treatment. If I look at a patient and ask myself Dr. Miller's question it makes all the difference in my approach to that patient's problem. If I view the patient as a complex system interacting with the environment, the difference is that I must do everything reasonable to help establish balance in the system.

Balance means providing all the necessary elements to optimize the system and removing any interfering elements. Nutrients are necessary elements. Toxins are interfering elements. The difficulty is that each of us is unique, and the necessary and interfering elements differ, sometimes widely, from person to person. In systems analysis, in treating each person as a unique problem what counts are the differences between that person and others. In traditional medicine, in treating each person as a disease it is the similarities that count.

As I am defining it, cyberhealth means understanding health as an ever-shifting state in the complex web of interactions which, when working in harmony, yield a dynamic balance that we experience as feeling well.

As is true for computers, cybernetics in biology can be grasped, even by the beginner, in terms of such certain recurring generalized functions as input, storage and output for a computer and perception, memory and language for a person.

When I finished my training and thought I could stamp out illness with my ballpoint pen and prescription pad, I was comfortable with the landmarks I had been given to find my way as a doctor. I had a detailed view of the real world inside the human body as well as an imaginary world populated by diseases whose attack I believed to be responsible for illness. A belief in that imaginary world works quite well in the management of the acute illness that one encounters in hospital wards where most medical training takes place, and the narrow path works quite well for treating trauma, acute infections or the intense phase of a psychosis. Belief in the same imaginary world did not work well for me as I entered family practice in a health maintenance organization, and patients began asking me questions that began with the word *could:* "Could my cramps and diarrhea be caused, not by colitis, but by something I am eating?" "Could taking vitamins help my depression?" "Could my child's hyperactivity be caused by allergies?" As I began to struggle with the answers to those questions in the spirit of Dr. Miller's question, "Have I done everything I can for this patient?" I began to leave the security of the narrow path, putting a tentative foot on the broad path of the systems approach to health. The first 10 chapters of this book tell the stories of patients who have helped me find security on the broad path.

As I have tried to sort out my patients' chronic illnesses over 30 years of practice, I have found a much more navigable and realistic terrain than the imaginary one I learned in medical school in which illness is seen as the attack of a disease. The landscape of cyberhealth is revealed in a functional, as opposed to an anatomical, view of things. Of all the various functions in human biology there is one overriding function that connects to all the others. Understanding its chemistry and immunology can unify the physician's approach to problems of any level of complexity. It is detoxification.

When I speak of detoxification, I do not mean a treatment for alcohol and drug abuse, although such treatments are tangentially related to the subject of this book. I mean the processes by which the body rids itself of unwanted materials. I do not mean what happens in the bathroom, whether that is bathing or emptying the bowels or bladder. I refer to the biochemistry of handling potentially harmful chemicals that appear within the system and which must be neutralized before they pass from the body. I am not referring exclusively to the harmful environmental chemicals we have all learned to fear: lead, mercury, other heavy metals, additives, dyes, hormones, pesticides, herbicides, fungicides and petrochemicals of all sorts or pollutants of the air, water and food supply that we ingest.

Detoxification is central to understanding functional assessment in medicine not so much because we live in a toxic environment but because detoxification is the biggest item in each individual's biochemical budget. It handles waste not only from the environment, but from every process in all the organs and systems of the body. Nearly every molecule the body handles has to be gotten rid of when it has served its purpose. Doing so involves a deliberate process of rendering the molecule inactive. It is a synthetic activity, a creative enterprise in which small molecules—such as the ammonia left over from protein metabolism, hormones no longer needed by the endocrine system, used neurotransmitters from the nervous system, or the byproducts of a well-functioning immune system—must be changed before they can be safely excreted from the body.

Illness and disease will affect the body's detoxification chemistry, and if there is something wrong with the detoxification chemistry, any other problems will be aggravated. It is central to all systems. Detoxification chemistry provides the map and the vehicle for understanding the functional landscape of each human being. It offers a new way to defend the body's health by establishing and maintaining a state of balance instead of waiting in fear for an expensive disease to strike. In fact, the conventional medical disease-oriented approach to health care is sinking the medical economy. We will not be able to save medical dollars until we change the way we think about illness.

You need not wait for public policy to recover from the collapse of the current health-care system to adopt practices based on a modern understanding of biologic systems. If you understand some basic principles, you can make choices that will reduce your risk of illness and enhance your health. In the chapters which follow, I will retrace some of the paths I have taken as a practicing physician. Then I will explore how the chemistry and immunology of detoxification unifies our grasp on health problems more effectively than just giving problems a name and prescribing pills to suppress symptoms. I will explain detoxification chemistry and the tests that can be used to investigate how yours works. The concept of toxin embraces a wide variety of familiar substances that may pose problems for some people and not others. Individuality is the key to this book. Taking charge of your own health depends on knowing how to assess your individual biochemical and immunologic quirks. This book is designed to help you by using the same method I use in my office, taking plenty of time to explain detoxification concepts and considering all the angles.

This book is a personal account. The practice of medicine is a personal activity in which I take responsibility for sifting and filtering scientific information for my patients just as I have done in writing this book. This is not a dispassionate and objective overview of biochemistry, nutrition, detoxification or any other branch of objective science. The older I get, the more convinced I am that much of science depends on personal viewpoints, if not on personalities. In these pages you will find facts and ideas that are not all mine, but their assembly is a reflection of my personal viewpoint as a practicing physician.

# Detoxification and HEALING

# CHAPTER 1

# The Unity of the Immune System and the Central Nervous System

IN EXPLAINING to my patients how I go about the detective work involved in unraveling their problems, I sometimes recite the "Tacks Rules" to make my point.

> 1. *If you are sitting on a tack, it takes a lot of aspirin to make it feel good.*
> 2. *If you are sitting on two tacks, removing just one does not result in a 50 percent improvement.*

Let's look at the first rule. You could substitute the word *aspirin* with *psychotherapy, meditation, organic foods* or *vitamins* and the rule still applies: the proper treatment for tack-sitting is tack-removal. Get at the root of the matter and fix it. In particular, don't take medicine to cover up a symptom instead of looking for the cause.

Chronic illness has two common roots, one of which is illustrated by the first rule: The body may be irritated by an unwanted substance. If not a tack, it could be a disagreeable substance such as a food that causes an allergy, it could be lead or a germ or a naturally occurring or manufactured toxin. The presence of some unwanted substance is a common root of illness.

The second rule helps explain what I mean by root. Becoming chronically ill usually results from a combination of factors. It is unrealistic to think in terms of a single cause when several factors inevitably contribute to a problem. It is especially unrealistic to recommend a single treatment to remedy a complex chronic illness when several factors deserve attention. The factors may have to do with the presence of an unwanted substance or the lack of a needed substance. The main focus of this book is ridding one's body of unwanted substances, that is, detoxification. As you will see, effective detoxification cannot work well without critical dietary substances. Complete avoidance of offending allergens or toxins is not usually possible. Good nutrition to supply individual needs for certain basic nutrients becomes a top priority in improving efficient detoxification mechanisms. The basic biochemical facts of detoxification are well-established. My job is to enable you to make sense of the facts, many of which you already know.

Look at yourself. Do you see any part of yourself that is the same as it was when you were a baby? No. You are different. Is there anywhere in your body where you can find a cell that is the identical, undivided cell present when you were first old enough to blow out some candles on your birthday cake? Before trying to answer that question, let me pose a related question: if you think back to your first remembered birthday, where did you put that memory so that it still evokes the candles, the cake, your playmates or some extraneous detail of the day? You did not put the memory in your fingernails, or your hair, or skin, or liver or heart. All the cells of such parts have long since been replaced. Granted each cell transmits a certain kind of memory to its progeny when it divides, but that memory does not have to do with birthday parties, it has to do with your ancestors. Each cell carries DNA encoding your ancestral memory. But each cell does not have encoded pictures of your little friend

Jeffrey spilling fruit punch all over himself and your new sneakers when you turned seven.

There are only two places in your body where there are cells which have remained undivided and unchanged except for aging. One place is your brain, where there are many cells that do not replace themselves, but remain intact from infancy until death. The other place is the immune system, comprised mainly of certain kinds of cells, called lymphocytes, which are spread widely throughout the body with certain strategic concentrations. Lymphocytes of the immune system arise from parent cells and then go on to live a life of days to months. There is a subset of lymphocytes that arise in the early stages of development from the same source as brain cells and, like certain brain cells, remain the undividing guardians of the persistence and the memory of our self. Look at yourself again. It is not obvious that your body contains two sets of permanent cells in your brain and immune system, nor is it obvious that your body is made up of cells. It is. 100,000,000,000,000 (100 trillion) of them. Life goes on in the cells. Each cell is a unit of life. All of the processes that you will contemplate in reading this book take place inside of cells or on the surfaces of cells within your body. You may remember hearing that cells multiply. It seems quite reasonable that a number as big as 100 trillion must be the product of multiplication. Not so. All cells come into being as the result of *division:* division of the first cell from which each of us originally derived. That cell, the fertilized egg, was lost as it divided into two cells which each in turn divided into two, which each in turn divided into two, and so on. But the continuing process of division does not go on indefinitely. As you developed, certain cells took on specialized functions: the capacity to remain as nerve cells or lymphocytes, the guardians of your essential self.

From the time the permanent cells established themselves during the early months of your existence all of the other cells of your body became, by comparison, relatively transient. Blood cells live three to four months. That is an intermediate lifespan between the short-lived cells of the surface of your tongue, subject to daily wear and tear and replacement, and the cells of your bones and other deep structures, that are replaced at a more leisurely pace. Whether it is sooner or later, however, the dying of each transient cell is the end of a life of service to the small minority of enduring and immutable cells.

Most of us have an instinct to protect our permanent brain cells, which, after all, have the conspicuous protection of our skull. We know that harm to these cells presents a completely different problem than, say, a broken bone or a tongue burned on a hot cup of tea.

We do not have the same instinct to protect our permanent lymphocytes. We are not directly conscious of their doings, and they are not as subject to the sort of collective slaughter that occurs with serious trauma or loss of blood supply as, say, in a stroke. If you become aware of the need to protect the health of your permanent cells, then you will need to learn ways to keep the cells as fresh and flexible as possible.

Caring for the transient cells of the body is also important. Cancer or the failure of a vital organ can arise in these cells and the injured cells often cannot simply be replaced. However, certain cells of the central nervous system and the immune system share at least one key attribute: an enduring presence in each of us from infancy to old age.

There are other features shared by the central nervous system and the immune system. The first such shared feature is memory. Memory depends on the persistence of permanent nerve and immune cells. It does not seem that brain memories are inside individual brain cells, so you might lose the recollection of your seventh birthday party or the candles or the cake with the loss of a particular cell. However, the capacity for memory resides exclusively in the two tissues of the body where the permanent cells reside, linking these two features (permanence of cells and the capacity for memory) in the brain and immune system. Another feature of both systems is perception. Without perceiving the world, there would be nothing to remember. The brain perceives the world with the senses: vision, hearing, taste, smell and touch.

Look at yourself yet a third time. You are perforated. You have a pair of eyes, ears, nostrils and a mouth by which you take in the world. Eating involves a very literal taking in of the edible parts of the world, but otherwise I speak of "taking in" the world of our senses when I perceive a friend's face in a photo on the wall of my office, the chirping of the chipmunks waiting for me to feed the birds, the scent of the garden or the feel of the keyboard as I write these words. The face, the phrase, the peonies and roses and the keys that I perceive this morning have been taken in without actually entering me. Their images have come to share residence in my enduring nerve cells, my central nervous system.

For example, while I was taking in the morning air I was also taking in something of which I was unaware until a sudden chain of sneezes left me incapable of attending to anything beyond the tip of my busy nose. What was that all about? It was a response to having taken in something that I did not take in with my conscious mind. Grass pollen grains on the morning breeze found their way to the mucous membranes of my nose where they were perceived not by my brain's senses but by my immune system. My immune system has remembered something disagreeable about grass pollen and was able to pick up the offensive taste or smell of it while my brain was happily focusing on the peonies and roses and completely unaware of the grass pollen. Then my chain of sneezes let me know that my old antagonist was getting to me. Without my conscious participation, my immune system has noticed and responded to particles that would otherwise be visible only to the eye aided by a microscope. My immune system has done something fully equivalent to the activity of my senses and my brain working together: recognition.

The main difference between the activity of my immune system with respect to the grass pollen and my brain with respect to the everyday world of my senses is a matter of scale. My senses and brain take in and remember, hence recognize, the big world of faces, peonies, roses, chipmunks and keyboards. My immune recognition deals with the invisibly small world of pollens, molds, germs and molecules. The chemistry of immune recognition is actually a lot like the chemistry of perceiving odors, and the chemistry of the immune system in general shares many of the molecules that carry out central nervous system function. We draw the line between the two depending on our level of conscious perception, and to a certain extent, on being able to identify the source of the odor with our other senses.

So far, I have made the point that memory resides in the central nervous and immune system, which are the home of the body's permanent cells. Now I am saying that the brain and immune system share another function: perceiving the world.

When we perceive things in the world of our senses, we are used to combining input from more than one sense to get the full picture of what is going on around us. We have a direct experience of the combined use of our senses. We do not need scientists to tell us that my experience of this morning's walk has required an overlapping, redundant collaboration of my vision, hearing, olfactory sense and touch to get me to my cottage. We do need scientists to tell us how the immune system carries out a similar overlapping, redundant collaboration of its perceptual faculties to form a picture of what is going on, not so much around, but in me. At its current state of development, immunology tends to view immune perception and memory in its particulars rather than in its combined effects. Major debates go on among scientists who have invested generous measures of ego in the importance of a particular immune mechanism in the detection of my offending grass pollen. My guess is that when it is all better understood, we will find that the immune system works very much like our senses and brain with respect to the combined, redundant and overlapping efforts of various "senses" required to identify and respond to our microscopic and molecular world.

Immune function and central nervous function are identical. Each perceives and each remembers. We use the word recognition with equal comfort in describing activities (perception and memory) shared by the brain and immune system. The only difference, except for anatomy, is the size of the objects we perceive and remember.

The only event I now remember from the first week of September 1960, when I first entered medical school, was my introduction to the corpse of a woman who had generously donated her body for my instruction. I cannot remember the location of my mailbox, my lecture room in public health, statistics or physiology or where I parked my car, but I remember every muscle, nerve and artery of the cadaver I shared with my classmate, Richard V. Lee. I remember the smell and the layout of the room, the location of our dissecting table by the door and the gradual revealing of the tissues' mysteries as I dissected day by day for nine months.

As I learned anatomy I also learned that my activities were part of a tradition that began during the Renaissance when medical scientists began the methodical dissection of cadavers. The arrangement and appearance of the internal organs, and later, their appearance under a microscope, formed the basis for understanding the workings of the body. Physicians who based their practice on such an understanding could claim a justifiable expertise gained from being able to visualize things that are ordinarily invisible.

Like pioneer anatomists and surgeons and like every other initiate medical student I tried to learn how the body works by exploring its details. My microscope took me beyond the sight and feel of the embalmed tissues. I saw how strikingly different the cells that form the tissue of the various organs appeared under the microscope. Muscle cells are long and slender, skin cells are flat like flagstones, cells that line the bowel wall are gobletlike cylinders and nerve cells have extensions so long that it takes only two cells to connect the brain and toes. It took a special insight for early histologists to realize that, however different, all tissues were divisible into the same basic subunit: the cell. The fantastic differences between the shapes of cells correspond to their varying functions. From that perspective the cells of the brain, with their long roots and branches, all consolidated in the head, seem quite alien to the cells of the immune system with their individually compact appearance and collectively scattered distribution in the body. It is understandable that the unity of the immune system and the central nervous system might be overlooked by anyone penetrating the body's mysteries with a dissecting scalpel, probe and microscope.

The medical sciences of non-European cultures did not rely on dissection as a way of penetrating the inner workings of the body. An accumulation of empirical evidence based on the testimony of living, not dead, bodies gave rise to an "anatomy" that seems quaint because its diagrams do not fulfill the eye's expectations based on surgery and dissection of cadavers. The diagrams may, however, present a picture of the dynamic balance among forces inside and outside the body that cannot be perceived in a cadaver. Neither

European traditions of anatomical dissection nor non-European empirical and contemplative traditions recognized the key notion that the immune system and central nervous system are in fact unified.

The immune system was the only part of my cadaver that I could not localize. I found the spleen, the remnants of a thymus gland beneath the breastbone, lots of insignificant appearing lymph nodes, and the place deep in the left side of the neck where the entire lacy network of the body's lymphatic vessels drains through a single passage into the subclavian ("under the collarbone") vein. Only in the last three generations have scientists understood how this system works at a cellular and molecular level, and only ten years ago did I first hear a professor of immunology (John Dwyer at Yale) state that the immune system and central nervous system share the distinction of being homes for cells that remain intact from infancy to old age. He and I and others of our generation in medicine, and you, perhaps, are startled to think that the immune system and the brain are really the same system. We have been schooled to think anatomically that these domains are quite separate. A "new discipline" of psychoneuroimmunology has grown up around observations linking the function of the brain and psyche with that of the immune system, which had been considered on anatomical grounds to be quite separate. For example, many individuals who have suffered the loss of a loved one undergo a period of immune suppression during the time of their most intense grief. As startling as the connections between the brain and immune system may be for those of us who have based our thinking on anatomy, we should not be surprised to recognize the immune system and brain as a unit if we base our thinking on function.

Taking a fresh look at human beings, an alien being might reasonably ask: "How does the human perceive the environment?" and "Where is the memory?" If such a being had the capacity to see that there are nests of cells in our bodies that are permanent while other cells come and go, it would see that these same cells are the basis for the functions of perception and memory; that they are the "essential" cells, the center of the abiding individual and the basis for the persistence of the self in a human being. The alien would reasonably assume that we human beings take special precautions to protect the vitality of our essential cells. Like queen bees, the irreplaceable and endangered essential cells of the immune and central nervous systems must be afforded a special degree of security, nutrition and respect.

If you, yourself, now realize that you have irreplaceable nests of cells that help you perceive and remember your experience of the world and that are the basis for the persistence of yourself, you may ask what needs to be done to ensure their vitality. At the very least you would conclude that your essential cells should have the best food and should avoid toxic substances.

# CHAPTER 2

# The Care and Feeding of the Permanent Cells:

## A Case of Infertility

How CAN THE ESSENTIAL permanent cells be protected? The following case history of infertility in an apparently healthy woman provides a model for looking at the health of cells.

Most of us have a direct experience with cells in the form of hen's eggs. I eat them for breakfast occasionally and recently I have become the beneficiary of a friend's hobby of raising chickens. Far from being a commercial operation, the hen house is a kind of poultry health resort which stops just short of providing manicures and massage for the hens. The children of the family provide love and attention to the hens, which are free to roam within the boundaries of their protection from coyotes and hawks. When I crack the white, brown or blue-green eggs into the pan the yolk sits up high and is a brightly glistening orange compared to the flat yellow yolks of the eggs from the supermarket. The eggs from my friend's hen house look so much better that no one could deny that they are healthier. I suppose that they are healthier to eat. It is reasonable to assume that the more fresh, lustrous and handsome our food is, the healthier it is to eat, so long as the food's appearance is not achieved by adding or applying toxic substances. I was thinking, however, about the better looking eggs from the hens' perspective and how egg appearance may apply to people's eggs. Assuming that the better looking eggs are healthier, from the functional (i.e. reproductive) point of view, it would follow that human eggs would look (and work) better if their bearers were well nourished and well cared for women.

When Sylvia Franco* first consulted me about her infertility problem, she had spent two years and more than $100,000 on infertility evaluation and treatment with all of the modern approaches, including a few attempts at *in vitro* fertilization. However, nobody ever asked her whether she ate well. She, a physician with a law degree and a master's degree in Business Administration, is a high-powered professional, a person for whom achievement had always come easily. Sylvia worked hard and had achieved a remarkable success in her early 30s. Her inability to conceive was the most bitter failure she had ever faced. She felt that not only her own previously trustworthy body had let her down, but also her own medical profession. She knew how to navigate the system and had seen the best consultants, but without success.

From my perspective, consulting about infertility is analogous to going to the doctor and saying, "I have these sets of permanent cells in my body, and I want to know if I am doing all I can to protect them and help them thrive. The person asking such a question may be in "perfect" health, as was Sylvia Franco. A natural beauty, she had always been healthy. Her 20-page medical history questionnaire was quite bare of details that might give me leads. She slept well, exercised and worked hard, had a good appetite, had no problems with her skin, hair, nails or respiratory, digestive or urinary systems. Her mood and energy were stable and she never had headaches or other aches and pains. She had had mononucleosis in college. After taking birth control pills for five years in her 20s her periods became light and then stopped just when she was trying to

---

* All of my case descriptions are based on factual experience with patients, with names and other identifying information altered to safeguard privacy.

get pregnant. Otherwise the only detail that attracted my attention was that she had a history of "bad teeth" with many cavities. She had taken antibiotics a few times in her life, but much fewer than most individuals whose parent happens to be a doctor. She had no history of yeast infections.

Sylvia and I agreed that her history provided only: 1) A small question about her nutritional status and the effects of birth control pills, which place a special demand on a woman's system with respect to several nutrients,[2] including folic acid, vitamin B6 and magnesium; and 2) Some room to speculate about her mineral status because of her poor teeth. Usually bad teeth have more to do with the flora and acidity of the mouth, but mineral nutrition is something to consider. Finally, anyone who has taken birth control pills and/or antibiotics should consider whether this has altered the flora of the intestine in a way that favors the overgrowth of yeast. Also of interest in solving this problem was the fact that Dr. Franco had always consumed a diet that was high in sugar. Thus she was likely to be deficient in minerals and other nutrients and at risk for yeast overgrowth.

My experience with infertility had taught me the value of looking beyond the reproductive system after the basic gynecological work-up proved to be normal. In Dr. Franco's case, the history was so devoid of clues that I thought a survey of her biochemistry might be helpful in turning up things in need of fixing. The approach in that domain would, I explained, be quite simple: find things that are out of balance, fix them and hope for the best. She and I had a common understanding of what "biochemistry" consists of. We only differed in our concept of how far one can take the study of blood, urine and so on to see how an individual may be out of whack. Physicians understand "chemistry screen" to mean a panel of tests that are routinely run to assure that a patient's liver and kidneys are working and that there is no major anomaly in the blood levels of the major mineral elements, such as calcium and salt. These are the kinds of tests that Dr. Franco and I learned in the last two years of medical school. In the first two years we learned about the fundamentals of chemistry as expressed in the balanced interaction of sugars, amino acids, fatty acids and about 20 mineral elements, some of which, like chromium, are present in the body in only very small amounts. Most physicians do not consider it worthwhile to look at the balance of such substances in patients or to consider individual needs for vitamins that function as workers on all of the assembly (and disassembly) lines where the sugars, amino acids and fatty acids undergo various kinds of transformation in the process called metabolism. Some physicians, like me, do.

Then there is stool analysis, which is not the preferred specimen in most conventional medical settings. A short premedical stint in Nepal and two years of doctoring in Africa provided me with opportunities to learn parasitology, which is the usual motive, other than a search for hidden blood, for asking patients to submit a fecal specimen. I have learned to revere the digestive, metabolic and microbiologic information contained in comprehensive stool examinations, so I asked Dr. Franco to submit the appropriate specimen to a lab that specializes in the analysis of an otherwise unpopular material.

The results of the various tests indicated that beneath Dr. Franco's healthy-looking surface there was a biochemical disaster area. Of course, if you do enough tests you can find something wrong with just about everybody. However, these test results showed far more than a random departure from statistical norms; they revealed a picture of inner biochemical and immunological imbalance that called for multiple remedies to bring Dr. Franco's system into better balance: getting more of the substances she lacked and ridding her body of substances that were impeding her fertility.

As described in more detail in chapter 15, tests showed abnormalities in the germs inhabiting Dr. Franco's intestines and irregularities in amino acids that play a key role in detoxification. Simple and non-toxic treatment of these conditions were associated with her becoming pregnant within a few months. Her eight-and-a-half-pound baby Danielle does not prove that the approach taken to her mother's chemistry and immunology resulted in Danielle's successful conception. Coincidence and destiny are both involved in reproductive events. Dr. Franco's attempts to repeat her first successful pregnancy using the same treatments have so far been unsuccessful.

Dr. Franco's experience is typical for men and women who have consulted me about infertility problems. Besides, this anecdotal case illustrates a kind of common sense imbedded in the question about how to know if the permanent essential cells (Dr. Franco's eggs in this case) are in an optimum environment to help fulfill their destiny. Common sense tells us that the essential cells, like Swedish ivy on a window sill, will do best if they are given the right amounts of the substances they need and are protected from noxious substances. There are tests to find out about these two facets of clinical strategy. The rest of this book will present an overview of how the body works so that you can understand tests that may be helpful in sorting out problems as well as the "do's" and "don'ts" found in many books about health. This book is more about "whys" and "wherefores."

CHAPTER 3

# Toxicity from Without:

## The Ambassador's Daughter

WHEN I LIVED in Chad as a Peace Corps volunteer in 1968 the capital (now Njemena) was called Fort Lamy. Fort Lamy was more of a capital village than a capital city. Seen from the air, it was a sprawling version of the mud brick houses found in villages scattered thinly across the part of Chad that enters and then occupies the eastern Sahara Desert. Except for periodic forays by truck to "the bush," as the countryside was known, to visit and supervise my covolunteer nurses and technologists in various population centers, I made my way around Fort Lamy on my bicycle, an unheard of means of transportation for any of the small contingent of foreigners living in Chad as part of the diplomatic, foreign aid and French military communities. None of the contingent of less than two dozen physicians in all of Chad, most of whom were French military, would be seen driving anything less than a Peugot or a Land Rover. My job was to look after Chadians and to lead our Peace Corps team of nurses and technicians. I was surprised, therefore, to have a messenger arrive at my gate late one evening with an earnest request from a large Asian nation's ambassador to Chad. His seven-year-old daughter, Sue, was acutely ill and I was asked to attend to her. As she had better transportation at her disposal than I did, it was arranged that I see her immediately in my cubicle at the Peace Corps office, which was a short walk from my gate.

Acute is an ambiguous medical term that can mean sudden, recent, and/or serious. The distinction between acute and chronic illness is not completely clear, but it is entirely central to many of the issues I would like to clarify in this book. Many medical practices that apply to acute illness are not appropriate when applied to chronic illness, particularly the belief that naming the problem is equivalent to understanding it. Some medical lessons learned from acute illness are, however, instructive in understanding the mechanisms that may lie beneath chronic illness. The lesson I learned from the ambassador's daughter still keeps me on my toes for any kind of illness I confront in my life as a physician.

The child was prostrate. Her condition was one of deep stupor combined with a high fever. Responsive to painful stimuli, but not apparently hurting in any particular place, she had become suddenly ill on the preceding day. Another physician had advised her family that it must be *un coup de paludisme* (malaria attack) which is the Chadian equivalent of the American pediatric refuge "it must be a virus," except that the advice comes with specific recommendations that various anti-malarial measures be augmented. Facing another long night with an increasingly sick child, the ambassador had called my ambassador seeking someone to give a second opinion. Ambassador Morris reassured him that my worst past indiscretion was having gone to Yale, where I was to return at the end of my Peace Corps stint from Chad to serve as chief resident in pediatrics. After Sue and her parents and I had settled down in a space that bore no resemblance to an examining room, I took a careful history, which turned out to be all too simple. Sue had been in robust health and protected by immunizations and regular malarial prevention medication until the day before. Since its onset, her fever and lethargy had been unremitting—unlike malaria, which usually gives a pattern of fever broken by sweats. She had not complained of pain and her bowel movements and urination, while infrequent, were otherwise unremarkable. She had had no respiratory symptoms and no family member or playmate had been sick. The most important question on my mind was, "What terrible disease *doesn't* she have?" Even if a patient is not worried about having an awful disease when consulting a doctor with a headache, abdominal pain or occasional numbness in the fingers, a doctor's first job is to rule out the worst possibilities: a brain tumor, an appendix about to rupture, multiple sclerosis. Once the worst possible considerations are off the list, then the more optimistic side of the detective work can begin.

I studied my patient as she was carried in. She was just aware enough of her surroundings to know she did not want to be there and gave me a meeching* look. Her skin was flushed and hot to the touch. Her temperature, taken under her arm, was over 104.7° (40°C). Meningitis or encephalitis rank high on the list of worst possibilities, so I started by looking carefully for evidence of these as I examined her optic nerves with my ophthalmoscope, checked for a lack of suppleness of her neck and spine, checked her reflexes and her muscle tone. She was weak but nowhere paralyzed. Encephalitis would have been the trickiest diagnosis to rule out on the basis of physical exam. I was prepared to do a spinal tap. Otherwise my technical and laboratory resources were limited to what I could do with my own senses, aided by my microscope. It took only a few minutes to complete my physical examination, which revealed absolutely no localized sign of an infection that could explain the girl's condition.

I began to discuss the next possible steps with her parents, and none of the choices were ones they wanted to consider. I explained that I had fervently hoped to find a treatable cause of her problem, such as an ear infection. Since the 1950s, when antibiotics brought quick cures for many infections, finding "something to treat" became almost more satisfying than being able to report to worried parents that it is "nothing serious."

When I was an intern and resident in pediatrics at Yale, the expression "midnight ear" summoned the ambiguities of finding "something to treat." It is midnight in the emergency room. You have been on duty since 7 A.M. and have 14 hours still ahead, some

---

* Meeching means a look that pleads "I am helpless, please do me no harm." Dr. Louise Bates Ames taught me this word, explaining that it is a good old New England expression.

of them, you hope, asleep in the emergency room on-call bunk. A cranky child with a history of congestion and a fever awaits your decision while his worried and weary parents pray that the young doctor before them knows what he's doing. "I can't find any specific trouble, and I think he will be just fine if you take him home and keep an eye on him overnight" is not nearly as good an answer to their prayers as "He has an ear infection, and an antibiotic should take care of the problem." Even if there is no specific treatment, a specific name is needed. If the doctor can name it, he can tame it, or at least that is a common fantasy. As a worried and weary resident I prayed that careful examination of such a child's eardrums would reveal enough redness to justify the hoped for denouement. An ear drum that was just red enough for weariness and hope to take it over the threshold to treatability was a "midnight ear." If a small heap of ear wax prevented the young doctor from easy visualization of ear drums the potential for frustration demanded a mature conscience. Should the wiggling child be tormented with attempts to clean the ear, with the attendant risk of scratching the surface of the ear canal? The resulting spot of blood coming from the ear canal, however medically trivial, could be horrifying to a fear-struck parent inferring that the young doctor, who seemed okay until a moment ago, had just perforated the child's brain. Such situations gave rise to a pediatric rule of doubtful accuracy, that a red ear drum is never found behind a wall of wax.

I had honed my skills at non-traumatic wax removal and I summoned my confidence in those skills as I began to discuss the situation with Sue's parents. They had watched me take extra time examining her right ear with my otoscope. Could the problem be there, they asked, hopefully. "I think not," I said, because I had seen enough of her eardrum to be pretty sure that an ear infection could not explain her serious illness. Most ear infections in a child her age would not produce an illness like hers, anyway.

As I spoke, I was still bothered by the dark brown smooth appearance of her ear wax. Oriental people tend to have flaky or dry ear wax, and when I was trying to see Sue's eardrum around the obstruction I theorized to myself that her fever had melted the wax into the brown bead that obstructed my view. I am not sure why I stopped theorizing out loud to the ambassador and his wife to re-examine Sue's ear. I guess I realized that I had never seen such smooth wax in any child's ear, no matter what degree of fever had been present, and the melted wax theory just wouldn't fly. I could imagine no relevance of the abnormal wax, but was reluctant to dismiss any unexplained detail.

I explained that there was still a chance that some redness of Sue's right eardrum lurked behind a dome of wax that had kept me from being able to see the whole drum, but in the urgency of the situation I really just wanted to buy a little time to collect my meager thoughts. I carefully inserted my otoscope and inspected the wax until it transformed itself into the body of an engorged tick. Sue had a tick in her ear! Now I had to deal with further uncertainty. I was already in doubt as to which of several options would be the safest course for Sue. Now I had to contend with the risk of getting side-tracked by the delay and potential trauma involved in attempting to dislodge a critter known for its tenacity and whose presence was likely to be completely irrelevant to Sue's condition. I imagined the consequences of spending precious time trying to get the tick out when I should have been doing a spinal tap or sending Sue to the hospital to be cared for. The ambassador and his wife were especially resistant to the latter option, because they knew that the needles used there were sometimes not properly sterilized.

I put some mineral oil in Sue's ear canal in an attempt to start the process of suffocating the tick while I pondered what to do. A spinal tap would have been much easier than trying to manage the tick with my head mirror and a pair of tweezers. I decided to go for the tick as I realized that there was at least a possibility that the tick was making Sue sick. Madame Ambassador held the lamp from which the light reflected from my head mirror into Sue's ear canal; the ambassador held Sue tightly and I prayed for a steady hand.

I had just completed six months of a residency in obstetrics and gynecology before coming to Chad. Perhaps the skills I had learned there would see me through this delivery. I lined up the beam of light with Sue's ear canal, drew a bead on the tick and then obscured my view as I inserted the forceps that I hoped would embrace the tick. No big game hunter in the wilds of Chad could have felt the thrill I experienced as I withdrew my instrument with the quarry intact. While Sue's parents and I shared the first moments of this small triumph, we all realized that now we must get back to the main business at hand. Scarcely had we retrieved our pre-tick seating arrangement when Sue stretched and sighed deeply. Within three minutes she roused from her stupor, left her father's lap and embraced her mother. Within 15 minutes her body temperature dropped. Within a half an hour we three astonished and relieved grownups ushered the smiling and chattering Sue to the ambassador's Mercedes Benz. She was back to her normal self. I was not. I was forever changed.

I walked back through my gate in the warm midnight air with the shrill sound of Fort Lamy's insects squeaking, chirping and singing in my ear, feeling the elation of a do-gooder who has done some good and pondering a serious scientific question: "What was that?" An extraordinary reaction to an ordinary tick bite? An ordinary reaction to a tick bite in an extraordinary location? Would you call the substance injected by the tick an allergen or a toxin? It was a variation on the theme of tick paralysis caused by several kinds of ticks around the world, particularly in Australia where they take a significant toll on sheep, who succumb to their paralytic bite. Sue had tick toxicosis, and the form her illness took probably had to do with the location of the bite. The substance in the tick saliva may be viewed as venom or as an allergen, since it evidently affects different individuals differently.

Sue's illness and the quick recovery impressed upon me a lesson I cannot ignore when considering the possibilities in any patient's illness: do not overlook the chance that a person may be having a peculiar reaction to something. Frequent findings of such "somethings" bring me back to the phrase my pathology professor, Avril Lebow, repeated like a mantra: "Illness results from the interaction between an etiologic (i.e., causative) agent and a susceptible host." Some people have peculiar interactions with etiologic agents that we would not expect to make a person sick. These experiences have changed me from a doctor who focuses on finding, naming and treating diseases to finding and treating the unique interaction between my patient as an individual and unusual toxins and allergens.

Individual is the key word. Each of us is different. There are more differences among individual humans than there are differences among other creatures of a given species.

Sue did not have a disease, even though there is a name for her condition. She had a quirky response to something the tick introduced into the skin deep in her ear canal. A disease is a concept we form about a group of ailing people who share common features. Acute illness usually fits into characteristic patterns so that we easily form a concept of the group features that encompass, say, chicken pox, or a cold, or an attack of kidney stones. In such cases human individuality becomes submerged beneath the more or less uniform effects that some germ or trauma evokes. As a physician I am expected either to name the problem or to eliminate several likely (and worrisome) prospects. It is like going to the woodshed with my flashlight to investigate an unexpected noise. I should return saying "It was a raccoon" or "I could smell skunk" and assume that I had eliminated the possibility of a prowler. Many acute illnesses fit their statistical images. They are as identifiable as a raccoon or a skunk glimpsed or sniffed in the woodshed. Most acute illnesses can be learned the same way a naturalist learns to identify robins and wrens or maples and oaks by a few identifying features. Sue's illness was not like this. It was very much the unique response of a particular little girl to a particular kind of tick injecting a particular something into a particular place in her ear canal. Another little girl, another kind of tick or another location of the tick would probably not have produced the illness that I saw.

Sue did not have a germ. For example, Lyme disease is transmitted by ticks who deliver a particular germ with their bite. The tick must be attached for several hours before it can inject the *Borelia bergdorfi* germ. After that the germ must multiply so that it may be hours before a noticeable redness appears on the skin and days or weeks before other manifestations of illness occur. I get tick bites from time to time working outdoors in our part of Connecticut, which is heavily populated with ticks. The bite may itch for days after removing a deer tick or dog tick from my skin, so I know that even when no *Borelia bergdorfi* germs have gotten into me, there was something in the tick's saliva that caused a little reaction. Sometimes, in me, as in many people, the skin returns to normal as soon as the tick has been removed. So if the "something" that the tick injected into Sue was not a germ, which would have remained after the tick was removed, and if it was like the substance that often gives me an itchy spot, how could she have reacted in such an extreme way? Whether you call Sue's reaction toxic or allergic, it planted a question in my mind that I now ask about each patient I see, even when I know the name of his or her illness: "Could some part of this person's illness be due to a toxin or an allergen?" The question that naturally follows would have been unanswerable in Sue's case, but is worth pursuing in individuals with chronic illness: "If there is a toxic or allergic component, why is this person unable to rid herself of the toxin or why is she sensitive to the allergen?"

Before moving ahead, let us review some of the main points that I have raised, which will be discussed further as we proceed. First of all, we need an approach to illness that goes beyond naming the illness and suppressing the symptoms with drugs or other approaches that fail to identify the cause. Secondly, the cause is not always simple, but can result from a complex interaction of different kinds of imbalances within an individual. The notion of balance includes *getting* the right amount of substances to satisfy our individual needs and *avoiding* exposure to substances that are toxic or allergenic. Achieving such a balance is relevant to the protection of a group of cells within one's body that are permanent and undividing and thus make up the essential cellular self. The cells in question reside in the immune and central nervous systems and, as such, participate in an individual's capacity to perceive and remember. Protection of these cells involves optimizing the function of the other transient cells of the body which, among other functions, rid us of potentially harmful substances. Dr. Franco's case reminds us that a simple approach to biochemical balance can have dramatic results, and the case of the ambassador's daughter reminds us that individuals can sometimes have very unusual sensitivities that need to be taken into account in solving their problems.

CHAPTER 4

# Toxic Hormones:

## A Boy with Breasts

NEWBORN BOYS AND GIRLS have breast buds resulting from estrogen hormones that have crossed the placenta from their mother. In boys the tissue disappears completely in the first few months of life. Occasionally a girl keeps a little through infancy and childhood until normal adolescent changes lead to normal breast development. Teenage boys may also develop breast buds when they are in the midst of the rest of their adolescent sexual development. They can be a source of embarrassment as well as fear and confusion even if the situation is carefully explained. Boys and girls each have a share of each other's typical hormones, and a slight excess of estrogen or an increased sensitivity of breast tissue to normal amounts of estrogen in a boy may lead to temporary breast enlargement.

I wondered about that connection 30 years ago when as a resident in pediatrics seeing patients in the outpatient clinic, I was consulted by the father of a six-year-old boy with breast buds. I figured that if a newborn boy or an adolescent boy could normally have breast buds, then, maybe it could be a normal variant in a six-year-old boy. That boy, Sean O'Malley, had breast buds that made him look as if he were beginning to develop breasts and had caused understandable alarm in his family. My own lack of experience with anything like this symptom in a boy his age led me to jump to the conclusion that he had an estrogen-secreting adrenal tumor.

I admitted him to the pediatric service, ordered the necessary scans, and got a loud scolding the next morning during rounds when the endocrine specialists came around to see him and he was already down in the X-ray department getting his scan. "Don't you know that there have been only 11 estrogen-secreting adrenal tumors in boys reported in all of the world's medical literature?" I had not known that. I took some comfort that my mistake had not caused anyone real harm, but the ridicule I endured before the other residents, nurses, interns and medical students was painful. The endocrinologists wanted him back on the pediatric floor immediately and recommended blood and urine levels of various hormones before any further steps were taken. A call to the X-ray department brought the radiologist to the phone. "This boy has an adrenal tumor, so we need to take a couple of more films before sending him up to the pediatric floor." The scans were completed, the surgeons were called, the situation was reviewed with Sean and his family and the next morning Sean went to the operating room, where estrogen-secreting adrenal cancer was removed. His breast buds disappeared within a few weeks and he remained well. The endocrinologists wrote him up and published the case report. I have learned more from my mistakes than from my achievements. Sean provided an opportunity for a little of both kinds of learning.

## LUKE'S STORY

Recently I was confronted with the same problem in an eight-year-old boy named Luke. When confronted by Luke's problem, I did not have the feeling that the story would turn out the same way as Sean's; his breast tissue was much less advanced. I was obliged, however, to eliminate the worst possibilities from his list and ordered the necessary hormone levels and scans. They were normal. The puzzle remained. Luke had already been under my care for other problems when the breast buds appeared. As it happened, just before his mother reported his worrisome symptom I had done a test of his liver's capacity to detoxify various unwanted substances in his body. Had I not done so, I would not have guessed that his endocrine problem might be caused by a problem in detoxifying estrogen. Plenty of boys have problems with detoxification, but I had not seen another case in which it results in breast bud development. On the other hand, such a connection is not unheard of. Men with liver disease, such as alcoholics, often develop breast tissue because they cannot rid themselves of the small amounts of estrogen that their bodies produce. Breast development in men with liver damage is, in fact, so common that I figured Luke's symptom could fit that model, given that I knew that his chemistry was somewhat quirky to begin with. I will return to wrap up Luke's story after the following point about detoxification.

*Detoxification* is what your body's chemistry does to rid itself of unwanted chemicals, whether the chemicals are left over from your own metabolism or enter your system from the air you breathe, the food and water you consume, substances you rub onto your skin or use to treat your hair or the toxins and allergens produced by the germs that inhabit your intestine. The word *detoxification* is also used to describe a treatment intended to improve or assist this process. Toxins are substances that are more or less harmful in small amounts to everyone. Allergens are substances which, in small amounts, cause harm to one person and not another. Sue's reaction to the tick bite illustrates that the distinction between toxin and allergen is not always entirely clear.

The biologic process of detoxification mostly involves synthesis as opposed to degradation. That is, if you want to get rid of a molecule, such as estrogen, your chemistry usually sticks another molecule onto it, making it bigger, but less toxic. "Packaged" in this way, the unwanted molecule is discharged from the body directly from the liver into the bile where it travels to the intestine and out, or the liver puts the package into the bloodstream where it travels out of the body in the urine via the kidneys. Some toxins, such as heavy metals, find their way out through hair and nails. A minor exit for toxins is through perspiration. For the most part, however, toxins are bundled for excretion from the body by a process that results in a bigger, not smaller package. I surmised that Luke might be having trouble with the phase of detoxification that deals with the packaging or conjugation of his estrogen.

I had done two kinds of tests on Luke's detoxification chemistry. Several months before, Luke's mother had sent his urine specimen to Dr. Rosemary Warring at the University of Birmingham in England. Dr. Warring is a pioneer in sorting out the connection between childhood autism and a weakness of one of the body's main detoxification systems. This system helps us get rid of leftover hormones, neurotransmitters and a wide variety of other toxic molecules. Some such molecules come from our own metabolism, like leftover hormones and neurotransmitters, and some come into us with our food or are made by the germs that live in our intestines. This detoxification system—phenosulfotransferases, or PST—seemed normal in Luke, but subsequently I measured other parts of his detoxification chemistry and found that they were seriously under par. I detected the detoxification problems at about the same time that the tests for adrenal tumors and serious hormone disorders were complete, including a careful physical exam in which I assessed his body hair (less than normal for an eight-year-old boy) and the size of his penis and testicles, which were notably small.

When I recommended a treatment with various supplements intended to help the conjugation phase of his detoxification chemistry I thought that a possible connection between his breast buds and underdeveloped genitals and his detoxification problem was quite speculative and after the scans and hormone tests proved normal, I was prepared to treat the problem with the reassurance that nothing really serious, such as a tumor, appeared to be the cause. I suggested supplements as a detoxification treatment simply because I wanted to do everything I could to improve this crucial part of his overall biochemistry. It was a matter of finding as many things wrong as could be found and fixing as many as could be fixed, as in Dr. Franco's case.

Within six weeks of beginning the treatment for his detoxification problem, he grew hair on his legs, his breast buds disappeared and his genital size became completely normal for an eight-year-old boy. Of all the various explanations—coincidence, placebo effect, improved detoxification of estrogens—for what brought about this sudden change, I believe it was detoxification that solved the problem.

Luke's story, however unique in my experience, provides a vehicle for understanding connections between toxins, detoxification and hormones that we hear more and more about but may otherwise have trouble understanding. There are, for example, some pesticides that mimic estrogen. In addition, meat contains estrogens that have been used to fatten animals. Exactly how each individual responds to exposure to pesticides and estrogens in our food supply must vary as each of us varies. For some of us, our detoxification chemistry is very likely to make all the difference between benign and deadly effects of hormones. I will return to this theme in chapter 12.

# CHAPTER 5

# Toxins from the Gut

I HAVE A SPECIAL INTEREST in airplane crashes because my father died in an airplane crash when I was 13 and my mother's only brother died in another plane crash when I was 12. My dad's crash was the first major plane accident in which there was a successful legal effort to prove that human error had been the cause. Years later a small settlement was shared by families and lawyers that pressed the case. When I recently heard in the news of an American Airlines jet that crashed on its approach to Cali, Colombia, I was intrigued that within days of the crash pilot error was cited as the cause. Then came the news that alcohol had turned up in the intestinal contents of the pilot. The final story was that the pilot had indeed made navigational errors, but the alcohol was present as a result of "natural processes" that occur after death. He had not been drinking. The alcohol, which was not a byproduct of the pilot's metabolism, did not leave his body in the process of decay. Nor is alcohol a part of any molecule that could release it after death. Thus, it could be mistaken for the residue of a gin and tonic consumed during life. But where did the alcohol come from?

**Fermentation.** Sugar is the common source of energy for all living things. When it burns clean and releases all of its energy, the carbon, oxygen and hydrogen atoms in the sugar become water and carbon dioxide. When we burn the sugar (glucose) that appears in our blood after we eat, the "smoke" that comes from that burning is made of water and carbon dioxide as is the smoke from a candle flame, a cigarette lighter or a municipal incinerator. The municipal incinerator may burn dirty, yielding a lot of soot and ash; however, when the body burns glucose, it is clean and simply produces pure water, pure carbon dioxide and energy. Even though glucose does not burn dirty, it can burn incompletely so that the sugar molecule is not broken down to its most fundamental components but rather, into pieces that carry two or three of the six units (carbon atoms) of which the sugar was made. The two-unit product is alcohol and the three-unit product is lactic acid, which is familiar as the sour taste in yogurt or sauerkraut. Both alcohol and lactic acid form in the living chemistry of germs but only humans can form lactic acid as a metabolic by-product. The intestinal contents of the body of the airline pilot contained alcohol because the germs normally present in the intestine went on to continue producing alcohol as they had done in life. The alcohol accumulated because the pilot's liver was not available to detoxify the alcohol as it was produced. He, like everyone, was making about half an ounce of alcohol in his intestines every day. He, like everyone, was taking this alcohol into his system until death extinguished his metabolic fire, but not that of the germs that lived in his gut.

In life, the burning of the alcohol results in its detoxification. It does not need a sticky carrier to get it out of the body. It goes up in smoke. One of the reasons it is toxic, however, is that it must be burnt. Unlike other foods, including the lactic acid found in foods, the body cannot treat alcohol as something to be saved for later and stored as fat. Another reason that alcohol is toxic is that it interferes with the chemistry of living things.

Alcohol exercises its toxic effects in a variety of ways. The pickling effect of high concentrations of alcohol used as antiseptics or preservatives gives an erroneous image of the way alcohol may affect a living cell in the concentrations found where germs have released it. In such concentrations as well as in concentrations found in the blood and tissues of someone drinking alcoholic beverages, alcohol interferes with many different enzymes. Enzymes are large molecules that embrace smaller ones so that the latter can be assembled or disassembled. Alcohol has a particularly bad effect on a group of enzymes called cytochrome P450 that are the main workers in the body's detoxification system. In this way alcohol can function as a sort of master toxin, enhancing the toxicity of all other toxic substances and even turning a relatively harmless substance such as the common pain reliever acetaminophen (such as Tylenol) into a poison by seriously interfering with a person's ability to detoxify the acetaminophen. Alcohol also interferes with the activity of key enzymes in the transformation of fatty acids into hormones as discussed in chapter 8.

Next time you go past the liquor store, replace in your mind's eye the sign that says "Peter's Spirit Shop" with one that says "Fungal Toxins Sold By the Bottle." Everything in the store was made by fungi. Wine, beer, whisky, vodka, sake, tequila and rum are all made by fermenting the sugars found naturally in grapes, grains, cactus or sugar cane. The kind of fungus used by vintners and brewers and distillers occurs naturally on the surface of the fruits of every plant found on dry land. Various species of the fungus are found in soil, in the air we breathe, and living on the moist surfaces of our body. The fungus stops short of completely burning its supply of sugar and forms alcohol, which it tolerates more than some of the other germs that might compete with it for space in nature. The fungus' self-protective knack for producing alcohol was domesticated by our ancestors about 10- or 12,000 years ago when someone discovered that grape juice would develop special properties when left in a jar with the lid on. Later on, someone discovered that wheat flour could be leavened with some of the residue from the wine-making process, and that subsequently the residue from the leavening could be passed on in the dough, some of which could be saved as a "starter" to make more dough. The particular fungus in question constitutes a large fungal family called *yeasts*. The ones we use for brewing and baking started out as the same one found in nature on the surface of grapes. Eighteenth century Dutch experimenters found strains of yeast that were more suitable for brewing and others that were more suitable for baking, and Louis Pasteur completed separation of yeasts that we now distinguish as baker's and brewer's yeasts. In baking, the alcohol produced in the leavening goes up the chimney during the baking process. With wine-making, it is the carbon dioxide that leaves the brew and escapes into the air, so that, with the exception of beer, champagne and other sparkling wines, the alcohol is retained within the beverage while the bubbles of carbon dioxide escape.

## When the Body Becomes a Brewery

It was champagne that brought down Angela Carino. Wedding champagne. After two glasses she began calling the mother of the groom a slut and threatened to kill the young man serving shrimp on a silver tray. After another half glass of bubbly fungal toxin extract she fell on her face into a yew shrub. Her son and three other men carried her 200-pound limp body from the scene and it took 16 hours for her to recover her senses and two weeks to heal the lacerations she suffered from the fall. Her reputation is still scarred. At one time, Angela had had a normal tolerance for alcoholic beverages. Then she had a stomach bypass operation after failing to lose much of her 300 pounds by less invasive methods including dieting. After the bypass procedure, she became an alcoholic. Her special relationship with alcohol is simple from one perspective: she shouldn't drink. However, she does drink, and the consequences are devastating. From another perspective, it is complex: she can manage moderate amounts of expensive champagne or a fresh wine made by her European brother-in-law. Her response to drinking a couple of glasses of Dom Perignon is pretty normal. However, if she drinks champagne priced at less than $10 a bottle, she turns violent at first and then sinks into a kind of stuporous, toxic impairment of brain functioning. Many of us experience a milder reaction that varies with the quality of the champagne, reminding us that it is not the alcohol but other components of the wine that can cause its immediately disagreeable effects. I like champagne, but if it is inexpensive it gives me a terrible headache, so I just say no.

After five years that have nearly destroyed her life, Mrs. Carino is in the process of learning that her operation turned her into an alcoholic. The operation did not change the amount she drank. It did not change her usually sweet and generous personality. It allowed her to keep her weight closer to 200 pounds and it did something to her intestines that drastically altered her response to alcohol. How so? She became more sensitive. She became sensitive to something more likely to be found in inexpensive champagne than in expensive champagne or some other wines. It has something to do with alcohol, but it is not only the alcohol. It is the "congeners" or substances other than alcohol that are produced in the process of aging and fermentation.

The ambassador's daughter was unusually sensitive to a tick bite in a way that had to do with the type of tick and the location of the bite. Luke was sensitive to a slight excess of estrogen caused by his body's failure to detoxify his own modest supply. This led to changes in his body that might not have affected another boy of the same age. Angela Carino's sensitivity is different. She went from having a tolerance for wine that was more or less like other people's to becoming peculiarly sensitive to it after her intestines were re-routed to send food past the point where it could be easily absorbed and turned into fat. Instead her food now gets used by a host of germs that inhabit a part of her intestine that would have previously been only thinly populated with germs. What do her germs do with the food? They eat it, or, more properly stated, they ferment it. After her operation, Angela developed a sort of brewery in her own intestines. The yield of her internal brewery is not only triggered by cheap champagne. It is produced by a mélange of unpredictable, more or less toxic products of fermentation that includes alcohol. Her detoxification chemistry now has to cope with a daily load of toxins that it never had to deal with before, and it can no longer handle the extra load of alcohol and its congeners. I will return to Angela Carino's story later.

Charles Swartz went to doctors complaining of neurological symptoms: inability to concentrate and episodes of appropriate behavior. The diagnosis was elusive until a blood alcohol level was checked and found to be elevated. Normal levels are nearly zero, but some people have trace amounts of alcohol in their blood produced by intestinal yeasts. His levels were similar to those produced by drinking alcoholic beverages, but he emphatically denied consuming any alcoholic beverage and he, like many alcoholics, was thought to be a liar. Further investigation showed that he was absorbing alcohol produced by yeasts in his own intestinal tract. These yeasts were rewarding their host for his hospitality by consuming sugars from his diet and converting them to alcohol. His case was widely reported[4] and became a source of inspiration to lawyers defending drunken drivers. Mr. Swartz's circumstances were unusual, however. He, like Mrs. Carino, had had intestinal surgery and he had lived in Japan, which was the presumed origin of the mutant yeast with a special capacity for intestinal alcohol production.

## ANTIBIOTICS AND YEAST OVERGROWTH

Charles Swartz and Angela Carino each had had intestinal surgery, providing an altered habitat for the germs which, in Mr. Swartz, consisted of some Japanese brewing mutants and in Mrs. Carino consisted of other factors that produced alcohol and other toxins that altered her response to drinking. A more common way to alter the germs of the intestinal tract is to kill large numbers with antibiotics.

Earl Knight consulted me with peripheral neuropathy after he had read Dr. William Crook's book, *The Yeast Connection*.[5] Earl was in perfect health when he consulted a physician at age 18 for his college physical. The examining doctor noted the pimples on Earl's back and face and suggested that he take tetracycline, the antibiotic most often used for treating acne. Earl took the antibiotic for three years pretty regularly, and the pimples diminished some, but not enough to persist with the treatment. When Earl stopped the treatment his acne flared and became a mass of cystic lesions on his face, back and chest that were still a major problem when he came to see me 19 years later. In the intervening years, and beginning at the time of the tetracycline treatment, Earl first developed a diffuse eczema with red, itchy, sometimes cracking and crusting skin eruptions on his entire body with intense localization on the backs of his knees and the crooks of his elbows. When the cracks became infected, the dermatologist gave him antibiotics. Earl also struggled with depression and fatigue. After reading books by Adelle Davis, he tried vitamin and mineral supplements, which actually made most of his symptoms worse.

Vitamin and mineral supplements may not make you feel better, but they really should not make things worse. The dangers of nutritional supplements are limited to rare instances of unwise excess or imbalance in the way they are taken. For the most part the body knows how to handle these substances, which, unlike drugs, are a familiar part of one's biochemistry and are not toxic in a wide range of dosages. Why is it that some people report a variety of unpleasant symptoms when they take supplements? Earl, for example, experimented with all sorts of exceptionally pure supplements and repeatedly found that some of the B vitamins intensified the disabling burning of his hands and feet for which he consulted me in 1988. His reactions to vitamins, even those that might normally be prescribed for treating peripheral nerve problems, were so severe that I was reluctant to experiment with injecting vitamins to see if a different route of administration would make a difference.

I put Earl on a yeast-free mold-free diet and prescribed medication to kill the yeasts in his intestines. After Earl's problem was under control, and his vitamin intolerance was still present, my assistant, Jayne Barese, suggested that we try injections of B vitamins. No adverse reactions occurred and the shots gave Earl a boost of energy. Earl's prior difficulty with vitamins illustrates a common problem signified by intolerance to vitamins. In nearly every case it turns out to be related to the mediation of germs inhabiting the upper intestinal tract. The germs get hold of one or another vitamin or mineral for which they have a particular affinity and celebrate by producing extra amounts of whatever toxins it pleases them to produce. The toxins, liberated in the intestines, either provoke digestive complaints or they are absorbed systemically where they provoke all sorts of symptoms, depending on the person. In Earl they provoked the precise symptoms of which he complained during several years of misery before Dr. Crook's book led him to me. His hands and feet were on fire most of the time. He had a sensation of numbness that was more like wearing heavy gloves than an absolute extinction of his sense of light touch, pressure, pain or finger position. He is a professional violinist, so wearing his neuropathic gloves was a special burden.

When Earl first consulted me he had already experimented with his diet along the lines outlined in Dr. Crook's book. He avoided fermented and leavened foods and other fare that is or becomes yeasty. Orange juice, like other juices one buys at the store, for example, picks up some of the yeasts that naturally inhabit the fruit's surface. During the preparation of the fresh juice or concentrates used in making commercial juices, the few yeasts that get into the juice to begin with multiply so that they become quite abundant in the finished product without causing noticeable fermentation. There is nothing wrong with having a few yeasts in our juice any more than there is a problem with inhaling the many yeasts and parts of yeasts and other molds that are present in the fresh air we normally breathe. Earl found, however, that his symptoms improved significantly when he avoided bread, vinegar, commercial juices, unpeeled fruits and leftover food. His fatigue, depression, rash, cystic acne and peripheral nerve symptoms got worse when he broke the diet.

It is rare for a person to actually harbor a strain of baker's or brewer's yeast in his or her digestive tract. Usually any yeast that is consumed live on fruit or dead in bread disappears during the process of digestion. Earl Knight's sensitivity to yeast in food was caused by the overgrowth of other kinds of yeasts that flourished in his intestines when other normal germs were killed by the tetracycline he took for acne. These yeasts probably existed in his digestive tract in normal quantities before he took tetracycline. With the antibiotic, they became so numerous they may have crossed the line from being normal intestinal germs to causing infection. The other species of yeasts that had become bothersome when consumed in food were not infectious, but they produced a toxic allergic reaction in Earl. When I encouraged him to continue his yeast- and mold-free diet and gave him medication to kill the yeasts in his intestine, nearly all of his problems cleared up except for a remaining intermittent sensation of tingling in his fingers and toes that may have been an acceptable disability in a non-violinist.

## A NEW LOOK AT THE YEAST CONNECTION

Before I met Dr. Orian Truss in 1977, I knew that yeast was a relatively innocent germ with a capacity for causing stubborn vaginal infection, often provoked by taking antibiotics. The prevailing medical opinion then, as now, was that yeast infections were associated only with superficial problems, most of which could be seen through a vaginal speculum. Yeast germs were thought to became truly infectious only in people whose immune systems had been injured by cancer chemotherapy or radiation or in babies who might get a thrush infection in the mouth even if they had not been given antibiotics. It is common knowledge that people can have strange reactions to germs, such as the allergic reaction to strep germs that results in rheumatic fever. I had not considered that the yeast germs that normally inhabit the intestines could constitute an allergen, however. I knew that people could have allergic reactions to foods, but I did not think of yeast and mold in food as high on the list of possible offenders as are egg, wheat, milk, soy, chocolate and seafood.

On the other hand, I had already begun to reassess my diverse experiences with yeasts. Before going to Africa in 1966 I had done part of a residency program in obstetrics and gynecology. In Africa I trained midwives and treated many gynecologic problems. Most of the women I saw had never taken any antibiotics. Yeast infections were rare in those women. In the United States, however, from the introduction of sulfa drugs in the 1930s and antibiotics in the 1940s, the incidence of vaginal yeast infections had risen to epidemic proportions, until today there are TV advertisements for antifungal treatments to be undertaken based on self-diagnosis. I also appreciated that one woman might harbor what seemed to be a very small number of yeasts when seen through a microscope in a drop of vaginal secretion and yet she would have tissues that appeared to be scalded by the infection. Another woman might have mucus that was loaded with the kind of actively branching yeast that are supposed to be the hallmark of active infection and yet she would be completely free of symptoms at the time of a routine examination for a Pap smear. Dr. Truss's findings helped me reexamine what I had been taught. I began to think about what I saw in my patients in a new way.

Dr. Truss had seen a number of patients in his allergy practice who experienced a dramatic remission of illness when he treated what had seemed to be unrelated symptoms of respiratory allergy with desensitization and avoidance of yeasts and molds. Following a trail that was indicated by his early patients, he accumulated a body of evidence over a 10-year period leading to the publication of his first papers and, in 1982, his book, *The Missing Diagnosis*.[6] One has only to try out his simple concept on a few patients, such as Earl Knight, to see how easy it is to spot and treat individuals who have been sick for years.

By the time I saw Earl I had been including Dr. Truss's concepts in my thinking about chronic illness for more than 10 years, during which time Dr. Truss and I had organized two international conferences on the subject. We had hoped to establish a dialogue between practitioners who, using the most benign kinds of intervention (a yeast-free diet and a trial of antifungal medication), could easily see results in their patients, and academicians, whose reverence for the established truth creates a skepticism that is invaluable to one's professional thinking.

There has always been a dialogue in my profession between empiricists and rationalists.[7] Empiricists are those of us who believe what we see and rationalists are those who see what we believe. It seems to me that the belief system of modern medicine has become something of a handicap in permitting us to see well. If this were not the case, Dr. Truss's theories would have gained widespread acceptance long ago. Instead many members of the medical profession stubbornly refer to the truth as that which is revealed in medical texts and editorials produced by committees and they fail to simply verify it with a few patients.

The two conferences we organized were intended to bring together a faculty of clinicians and academicians and an audience of clinicians anxious for guidance on how to help patients, many of whom had diagnosed their own problems as yeast-related with the help of Dr. Truss's book. The first conference, held in 1982 in Birmingham, was a success, particularly because it brought about a respectful dialogue between clinicians who had direct experience with patients who had convincing histories and responses to yeast-free diets and antifungal therapy and academicians whose experience tended to be more focused on hospitalized patients with yeast problems. The second conference, held in San Francisco in 1985, was well-attended, but was disappointing because two of our main speakers canceled at the last minute. They were pressured to stay away by the organized opposition of a major medical society which denounced the yeast idea as heresy, partly because of rivalry with an organization that cosponsored our conference and provided continuing education credits for attending physicians. Leaders in infectious disease and immunology have since retreated from their strong denunciation of the ideas put forward by Dr. Truss, but some of the public statements and editorials of the 1980s are still quoted by various authorities to threaten the livelihood of physicians who treat patients with yeast problems and to deny insurance reimbursement for such treatment on the grounds that it is not medically sound. In fact, there are groups of doctors in various states who fancy themselves "quackbusters" and go after the licenses of colleagues who treat patients with yeast-free diets and antifungal medications.

Much of the credit for bucking the tide of orthodox medical opinion regarding yeast goes to Dr. William Crook, whose wit and sincerity have disarmed many skeptics to the point of at least acknowledging that there might be such a thing as yeast problems. He organized the very first yeast conference in Dallas in 1980, attended by a couple of dozen of Dr. Truss's first converts. Soon Dr. Crook was turning out books which have sold widely and spread the word among many people who would otherwise never have gotten help. His free and easy enthusiasm has infected a few academics, but for the most part the medical schools and drug companies have turned a deaf ear. One of the major manufacturers of antifungal drugs has recently started funding some research, but the others have stonewalled efforts to conduct research while enjoying the profits from antifungal drugs.

# CHAPTER 6

# Food as Toxin

LYDIA DVORAK WAS a fellow member of the Yale Medical School faculty, but I probably would never have met her if she did not live across the street. In the 25 years that have elapsed since the time of the story I am about to tell she has become a full professor and a leading expert in her field of psychology and molecular biology. When we were both junior faculty members and she and her husband came over for dinner she told me her headache story. She was pregnant with her first child and had developed, for the first time in her life, absolutely crushing headaches. They were the kind of headaches that left her basically unable to leave a darkened room and were literally blinding, with partial loss of vision. The nausea and vomiting that accompanied the headaches did not seem to have to do with morning sickness, but felt to her as if she were trying to eject some kind of poison from her body. Her obstetrician delivered the children of many Yale doctors and other professors, including my own first child, and was a particularly thoughtful and skilled doctor. After carefully listening to Lydia's story he identified her problem as migraine and implied very strongly that having a Ph.D. and a baby might be producing some inner conflict that expressed itself as headache. Lydia responded with a strong expletive, fled the doctor's office and headed two blocks down the street straight to the medical library. Even in those days, before computer searches, she turned up the literature on food migraine within a couple of hours and came up with her own diagnosis. She immediately abandoned the New York State cheddar cheese habit that she had acquired for the sake of getting good protein for her fetus, and her headaches stopped.

There is nothing wrong with New York State cheddar cheese. That is, unless you happen to share Professor Dvorak's sensitivity to tyramine, a natural substance produced in the aging of various cheeses and other foods such as red wine and chocolate. Sensitivity to tyramine is just that, a "sensitivity," not an allergy. This is, in my opinion, a silly distinction that still carries a lot of weight in my profession. In general, doctors take sensitivities quite seriously. They are especially careful about drug sensitivities or allergies. However, many doctors, like lay people, are very skeptical about food sensitivity.

## I Become a Believer

Milton Senn was chairman of the Department of Pediatrics and director of the Yale Child Study Center when I first met him. I was an undergraduate at Yale and lived in Davenport College, one of the residential colleges where faculty members might meet with undergraduates over lunch. Dr. Senn was a large, gracious man of Scandinavian origin with bushy eyebrows and a gentle warmth that babies could recognize at a glance and which seemed unsuited to the highly competitive medical school faculty where Dr. Senn thrived. Dr. Senn retired just before I became an intern in pediatrics, which did not inhibit me from seeking his advice and friendship, especially years later when I was asked to become director of the Gesell Institute. Dr. Senn had replaced Dr. Gesell at the time of Dr. Gesell's retirement from the directorship of the Yale Child Study Center, and Dr. Senn had taken that institution on a new, psychoanalytically oriented path.

When I was asked to direct the Gesell Institute, I asked Dr. Senn's advice and he gave his blessing to my effort, even though it was clear that I would continue the Institute's orientation toward biological aspects of development, even expanding the notion to include a medical practice that included adults as well as children. A few years later Dr. Senn became my patient and, in the course of taking his history, he told me the following story.

Not long after coming to Yale Dr. Senn and his wife consulted their pediatrician concerning problems their baby was having with her skin, sleep and mood. Dr. and Mrs. Senn were quite convinced that the baby was allergic to eggs. Her problems were severe, though she didn't eat large amounts of eggs. The pediatrician was skeptical and expressed some impatience that a professor of pediatrics and chairman of the department, for that matter, should entertain such a diagnosis as a hidden egg allergy. "Actually," said Dr. Senn at the time of their consultation, "we think she is so sensitive that she cannot even be tested." The pediatrician said "Nonsense," or words to that effect, and proposed an oral challenge of a small amount of egg. The amount was negotiated so that the resulting quantity was one-eighth of a teaspoon of egg white diluted in a quart of water, of which a teaspoon was offered to the baby. Shortly thereafter, she came within an inch of dying from anaphylactic shock. After she was resuscitated the pediatrician conceded that she was, indeed, a very allergic child.

Here was a stimulus quite different than a tick bite in the ear canal, a reaction to poorly detoxified estrogen, the negative effect of alcohol or other yeast toxins in a person with altered gut function or flora or the quirky toxicity of tyramine in cheddar cheese. This was just the tiniest bit of a perfectly healthy food, and it was nearly as lethal as the most toxic of substances. How can one person be nearly poisoned by a food that nourishes another? The whole process is so mysterious and physiologically perverse that it gets pushed aside in the training of doctors, who prefer to deal with situations that they can control. In my own training, my chairman (Dr. Senn's successor), Dr. Charles Davenport Cook, took a dim view of allergy and discouraged me from taking any interest in it whenever the subject came up of my own severe allergy to cats. Dr. Cook did encourage me to be interested in nutrition, but allergy was not considered a respectable pursuit. The pediatric allergy clinic at Yale was the only specialty clinic that was still under the leadership of practicing pediatricians from the New Haven community as opposed to full-time academics who, by the early 1960s, had come to dominate medical education in all of the major medical schools.

Except for the little I had learned from my own suffering with hay fever and cat-induced asthma, I knew little about allergies. I completed my training in pediatrics and, after a year as chief resident at Yale, I spent two years on the full-time faculty as an assistant professor of Medical Computer Sciences working in the Department of Obstetrics and teaching in pediatrics. When I went into practice in 1971 as a family practitioner and pediatrician, I believed that allergy, especially food allergy, was inconsequential and that lack of knowledge of it would not affect my ability to do everything I could for my patients.

I started out as one of four primary care physicians in the first Health Maintenance Organization in the Northeast, before the term HMO was in use. At the time we had to be fairly well-staffed even though patient enrollment was just beginning, so I had plenty of time to spend with patients, a habit that remains the backbone of my practice. Frequently, during relatively unfocused conversations with patients I learn helpful clues that open new avenues for solving their problems. I listen a lot. I take complete medical histories of the kind I was taught to do as a medical student and intern. Medical students (who work on the medical wards of the hospital as "clinical clerks") are required to write up a complete history and the findings of a complete physical exam of patients assigned to them when they are admitted to the hospital.

However it is organized, the traditional content of the history is supposed to begin with a statement concerning the presenting problem, usually quoting the patient's own words to describe what is wrong after a terse demographic statement: "Mrs. Smith is a 37-year-old, divorced, white paralegal and mother of two children who presents with "severe headache." After a description of the onset, duration, periodicity, aggravating and alleviating factors and associated symptoms the medical student is expected to record past illnesses, past injuries, allergies—especially to medications, drug usage, social and family history, and what is known as a review of systems, an inventory of complaints referable to the respiratory system, digestive system, reproductive system, etc. As the student progresses up the ladder, and eventually becomes a physician in his or her own office he or she generally adopts the hasty, illegible and incomplete methods of the top of the hierarchy.

Dr. Lawrence L. Weed, now an emeritus professor at the University of Vermont Medical School, came along in the 1960s to take some initial giant steps in teaching changes in record-keeping as well as the thinking that goes with it. The method in place at the time was to cap the history and physical exam described above with a discussion of the differential diagnosis in which the student explicitly describes his or her choices among the various diseases that could be present considering the history, physical findings and initial laboratory results. The value of the exercise is in helping the student learn to discard the irrelevant and focus on the relevant facts in arriving at a parsimonious conclusion concerning the patient's condition. Dr. Weed wrote and spoke eloquently and, at times, scathingly about the tendency of the diagnosis-oriented approach to overlook problems that were either important to the patient's overall health, e.g. getting divorced, or could have crucial ancillary importance to the treatment of the present diagnosis, e.g. underlying diabetes. His problem-oriented approach encourages physicians to list all the patient's difficulties, abnormalities and situations that can be described as problems without having to dignify them as diagnoses. The approach leads to thoroughness and it particularly discourages the medical tendency to lose track of details in a patient's story that are deemed irrelevant because they do not constitute criteria for arriving at a diagnosis.

As I learned a tolerance for tracking "irrelevant" details, I also learned patience with "irrelevant" questions posed by patients as they struggled to sort out the meaning of problems seen from their perspective. Such questions usually begin with the word "could."

When I started out low in the hierarchy as a Primary Care Physician—or "provider" as we are now called—I was particularly troubled by my patients' questions that began with the word "could." The more time I spent listening to my patients' stories, the more trouble I had answering with the time-saving word "no" that would be easier to utter if I were focused on making a diagnosis rather than on understanding all the problems.

The questions often came up when I was trying to take a complete medical history including, "Tell me about past illnesses, injuries, allergies, occupational exposures and medications you have taken." More often than I expected, my patients indicated in their reply to the allergy query that there were foods they avoided in order to prevent symptoms. Often patients had suffered for an extended period before making the connection between the foods they ate and their symptoms. If I had just heard that a patient avoided foods from the nightshade family (tomato, potato, peppers, eggplant, tobacco) in order to remain free of joint pain, I wondered what to tell the next patient who asked, "Could my joint pain have anything to do with my diet?"

The stories I heard came from completely reasonable and sane people, and when they differed from pronouncements in heavy medical texts that said, for example, that food allergies are rare, I tended to believe the collective voice of my patients. The more I believed my patients, the more difficulty I had giving a flat *no* to questions for which the answer might better be, "It is not likely, but it is possible, so we should check it out." Sometimes, the way to check out the likelihood of allergy was pretty obvious. For example, Hillary Tuckerman became wildly hyperactive when given ampicillin for her earache. Giving an antibiotic to a nine-month-old infant usually relieves pain very promptly.

I had never heard of ampicillin causing an infant to climb the walls, yet Mrs. Tuckerman said that Hillary had turned into a "wild raving animal," screeching and clawing the air, her bedding, her hair and her mother about an hour after getting her first dose of the drug. Roused from sleep in my on-call room I was faced with Mrs. Tuckerman's question, *"Could* Hillary be having a sort of psychotic reaction to the penicillin?" One thing I knew was that the family of penicillin drugs did not cause psychotic reactions. There is a temptation to stop listening when you think that the patient's question seems irrelevant. I had, however, long since learned to weigh the short-term rewards of the pillow against the greater rewards of careful listening. This I did as Mrs. Tuckerman speculated, "Could it be the pink stuff they use to color the capsules?" I didn't think so. "They"—the pharmaceutical company—surely knew how to make children's medicine and would not put anything in it that would turn Hillary into a "beast." "Still," Mrs. Tuckerman suggested, "There is Dr. Feingold who says that food coloring can bother some kids, even make them hyper." I had heard of Feingold, but all I knew was that he had written a popular book saying things that were not medically true. At the time I did not understand the distinction between *True* and *true*. It was probably two years after my nighttime conversation with Mrs. Tuckerman, while having tea served by Dr. Feingold in his 11th floor studio on North Point overlooking San Francisco Bay, that the difference between *True* and *true* really sank in.

Something is *true* when reasonable people examine the evidence with an open mind and, well informed of all the facts, admit that, for example, some children react to some foods or food additives with changes in mood, behavior, affect or attention. It took only a few minutes of conversation with Dr. Feingold for me to discover that he was a man of vast clinical experience: nearly 50 years of observing the effects of allergy. He had a critical mind and the forthright approach to saying what he had to say that is often found in people over 70 years old. A small, salty, agile man with generous eyebrows and a direct gaze, his conclusions, based on decades of experience, seemed so obviously reliable that the benefit of acting upon his truth (that is, suspecting reactions to foods and food additives when the possibility arises) seemed to me to clearly outweigh the risk of ignoring it. His truth has, however, taken a beating on its way to becoming the Truth. He did not publish his research results in a peer-reviewed scientific journal before writing a book that mothers brought to their pediatricians' offices as if it were a missionary's bible wielded before the heathen. Committees, editorials and grand rounds presentations denounced Dr. Feingold's description of reality, and eventually studies were conducted to "prove" that he was wrong. While the studies consistently turned up evidence to support his contention, they were published under titles and reviewed under headlines that touted "negative results,"[8] meaning that any doctor who chose to ignore Dr. Feingold's notions would have the protection of his colleagues and anyone who asserted even the partial truth of his observations would be considered a heretic.

My experience with Hillary was one of several at that time that helped me reconsider some of the dogmas of my mainstream training.

I had Mrs. Tuckerman come to the clinic where I took capsules of ampicillin and showed her how to open them and shake out the white powder so Hillary could take it with a little honey or applesauce as a substitute for the pink suspension. Hillary soon recovered from her earache without any side effects from the drug. Several months later I got a call from Ohio, where Hillary and her mother were visiting Hillary's grandparents. Mrs. Tuckerman wanted my help because Hillary had again been stricken with an earache. She had been seen by a Dr. Stone, an Ohio pediatrician, who insisted on prescribing a pink suspension. Mrs. Tuckerman had told the doctor about Hillary's previous experience and expressed her concerns about dyes and other food additives, but, according to Mrs. Tuckerman, the doctor ignored her and, with a roll of his eyes, pronounced, "Oh, that's Feingold." Reluctantly, Mrs. Tuckerman agreed to have Hillary take the prescription, and the results were just as she feared. Now the distraught parent wanted me to intervene and persuade Dr. Stone to prescribe an alternative for her daughter.

Calling Dr. Stone would not be easy for me. I learned Hillary's grandmother and Dr. Stone's mother played bridge together, and that Dr. Stone had been especially kind—getting up at night to actually observe Hillary in orbit. He had been as adamant about his views as he had been sweet to Hillary, and I did not relish speaking with him. I don't like calling strange doctors. I have had some exceptionally bad experiences even though the typical call often works out quite well, more so in the last few years as some doctors have become more tolerant of nondrug approaches to illness. However, at the time of Mrs. Tuckerman's call years ago, I was less experienced and more likely to be scorched by my colleagues' disaffection. The call to Dr. Stone went something like this:

"Hello, Dr. Stone. My name is Sid Baker. My patient, Hillary Tuckerman's mom, asked me to give you a ring. She is very grateful for your care of Hillary, but she is concerned about the possibility that the red dye in the ampicillin is causing a problem. I . . . ."

"Well, Dr. Baker, I appreciate your concern, but I think we

agree that Mrs. Tuckerman is a little overboard with this Feingold thing. I am a pediatrician, so I feel qualified to call the shots at this end," said Dr. Stone, who had taken the term "family doctor" as applied to me by Mrs. Tuckerman to imply that I was not a specialist in his domain. The soft gravel in Dr. Stone's voice let me know that I was speaking to a much older doc than me and one with whom I would have cordially agreed on the importance of breastfeeding or exercise, but we were not to reach agreement on the possibility of individual reactions to food colorings in children's medicines.

He protested by adding, "I'm a small town doc but I practice scientific medicine. I can't get carried away with every new fad, especially one that is not only unsupported in the peer review journals, but actually has been disproved, according to what I read. I have people here telling me that food colorings, salicylates and all sorts of other stuff cause this hyperactivity thing, and I just don't see it." Dr. Stone held to the same dogma that I was beginning to shed: Diseases are entities (e.g., "this hyperactivity thing"), and the clinician's job is to identify the disease and then aim therapy at it. If hyperactivity is the "thing" and "they" (peers) say that it is not caused by food additives, then a good doctor waits until "they" figure out what "the treatment" should be, meanwhile resisting any secular challenge to the whole idea of how people get sick; they are the victims of the attack by diseases. I could tell that Dr. Stone was going to yield on the case in point without ever yielding the high ground he had claimed. That was fine with me. I just wanted to get off the phone without having to call Mrs. Tuckerman with news of my defeat.

"Please understand, Dr. Stone, that Mrs. Tuckerman just thought it might be helpful for you to hear from me that Hillary had an identical reaction to the ampicillin that I prescribed for her and she cooled off as soon as we switched to powder from the capsules."

Tension mounted as Dr. Stone pointed out that I had probably not seen this "cooling off" with my own eyes, but, with the last word, he agreed that Hillary could have the capsules.

## A RESISTANT MEDICAL COMMUNITY

In those days I would actually seek out my colleagues at Yale and in the New Haven community and tell them about cases like Hillary's, figuring that my stock was high enough with them to put me on a different footing than I was in conversations like the one I had with Dr. Stone. Within a few minutes of starting such a conversation, however, my colleagues would talk about whatever "disease" my patient had and how there is not any "scientifically credible published" support for the notion that such and such disease is caused by whatever it was that affected my particular patient. I tried to return to the dialogue by saying "Look, this happens. For the sake of argument, accept the fact that on an individual basis patients have peculiar reactions to all sorts of things. Let's talk about how we might apply that to the diagnosis of patients with complex problems that may or not fit into some particular diagnostic category, but who may have some symptoms provoked by allergic or toxic exposures." I didn't succeed.

My colleagues, especially some of those with the best qualifications, were trained to win arguments. Their most successful tactic is to keep the discussion focused on "the treatment for the disease" and not to accept, for the sake of argument, a shift to observations that could be dismissed as anecdotal. I avoid such conversations now.

The case histories I've recounted are intended to prepare you for a discussion of the "whys and wherefores" of illness. If you understand some basic immunology and biochemistry, you will be better prepared to evaluate the kinds of tests and treatments that your medical doctor, nutritionist, psychiatrist, acupuncturist, personal trainer, coach, homeopath, naturopath, chiropractor, dentist, psychologist or sister-in-law may recommend in the name of good health. It is not likely that you will be bitten in the ear canal by a tick, but it is certainly possible that some critter, allergen, toxin, bacterium, fungus or virus will cross your path and lead you to ponder your options for preventing or alleviating the consequences.

You may need special lessons to make wise choices among your options when you are told to avoid fat, take antioxidants or minerals, avoid pesticides, hair dye, sugar, coffee, air pollution, medications, sunlight, indoor air, outdoor air, meat, wheat or long walks in the rain. If you develop chronic or recurring symptoms and wish to be an intelligent participant in your own detective work to sort it out, you definitely need special lessons. The lessons I have to offer will provide a point of view as well as some general principles of immunology and biochemistry that every adult should understand.

A particular point of view and a few basic facts are necessary to understand the threats whose combined effects on your body are usually described as a "disease." Understanding how your body handles the substances that enter it is a good place to begin our lessons about the true causes of disease.

CHAPTER 7

# You Are *Not* What You Eat

YOU SHOULD NOT GET "eggy" from eating eggs. If you eat an egg your digestive processes should remove the egginess from the egg's materials so that they enter your bloodstream stripped of any fowl identity and become available for you to impart your own identity on to the stuff that constitutes an egg. Ego is the name of the identity that distinguishes you as a unique creature. When your digestive process works properly it achieves a triumph of your ego over the substances you consume. Otherwise you would accumulate foreign materials whose presence in your structure would undermine your claim to exclusive dominion over your flesh. Not that you would become some sort of omelet of the remnants of your cumulative meals, but your body would be ever less purely "you." You might imagine that Mother Nature would save all of her creatures a lot of work by providing for a certain number of interchangeable parts so that molecules that are costly to synthesize could be moved from prey to predator and save the whole system the expense of their repeated disassembly and reassembly. Instead the system honors individuality so that even cannibal critters must convert their prey into small change and reconstitute the molecules from scratch. The small change is what we call "essential nutrients" and consists of very small molecules called fatty acids, amino acids, vitamins, minerals and accessory nutritional factors. If you were to apply the structural analogy to your dwelling, then the construction materials delivered to the building site would be sand or equivalent-sized particles of clay to make cement blocks and bricks, sawdust to make wood and iron filings to make nails and other metallic parts.

The arrangement—the complete digestion of all the food we swallow—does not always work as it should, so that, in fact, you might get a little eggy each time you eat an egg. It is not just a question of accommodating some vague essence of egg or even the less subtle taint of garlic that enters with your meal and leaves an odor on your breath. Some major molecules—composed of anywhere from two to thousands of subunits—escape digestion, enter your blood and have to be eliminated. A medium or large molecule that retains its egginess presents a job that is parceled out among functions that include sniffing, identifying, tracking, killing and disposing of it. So it is with all intruders, be they chemicals, foods, germs or the toxins produced by germs.

Smell or taste is a first test of a food's edibility. We may develop tastes for certain things, like Stilton cheese and whole fresh fried clams from the fish place down by the wharf, in spite of their unpleasant smell or off taste. For the most part, however, taste is your body's first and conscious effort to identify molecules that may cause mischief and to avoid them. Sometimes the taste is on the edge of acceptability, as was a mouthful of fried clam I purchased in hurried hunger at the end of a long and busy Saturday and brought home to be savored with homemade fixings and a bottle of red wine. "That last mouthful of river bottom belly of a big juicy clam was a little below standard," said my palate. But it was too late now that I had swallowed it. Or was it? Would the taste buds of my stomach give a second opinion? I spent the evening as a spectator to negotiations that were signaled by successive waves of satiety, discomfort, queasiness and nausea, and I went to bed to sleep it off. Our livers work on the night shift. I knew that as I prepared for bed my intestines were asking my liver to taste the clams to see if some accommodation could be worked out. An hour later I was awakened with a strong impression that my liver had come to a decision. The clam was going to be ejected, and my whole meal and beverage selection was going with it. The reverse peristalsis that followed was one of the most efficient operations I have ever witnessed in my body. All my efforts to learn to pole vault or throw the javelin for my track team were miserably awkward compared with the muscular expertise with which my stomach rejected my evening feast of clams and wine with a green salad and French fries.

My palate, stomach and liver had all tasted the bad clam. My mouth said "ugh" but the clam was not bad enough to spit out. My stomach said, "Let's put this and everything that came with it on hold and see if the liver can handle it," for nearly everything *except* fat passes through the liver—the next stop after the stomach and small intestines. The liver said, "I hate to sacrifice all those good calories, but the molecules in the bad clam are going to cause mischief somewhere in the body unless I can detoxify them and I can't." Note that the liver's job was *not* to decide whether the toxins in question would cause cancer. Nowadays when we hear about the safety or toxicity of potentially noxious substances, they are often judged good or bad depending on whether they can be said to cause cancer. That is not the liver's immediate concern when evaluating spoiled food. The liver has to decide whether the toxins would interact badly with any tissue or organ in the body, assuming the liver cannot find a way to deactivate the harmful molecules. This is a particularly delicate assignment when the bad molecules closely resemble good ones. As in all of nature, mimicry is a good way to escape detection; in the case of the bad clam its taste was just a little less acceptable than the ocean bottom taste of acceptable clams.

## How Foods Become Toxic

Before tackling the question of how spoiled foods harm the body, which will lead to a discussion of how we can and cannot protect ourselves from them, we need to consider how the bad clam and other "bad" substances become toxic. In the case of the clam, it became toxic after it died and it was dead too long when it joined the rest of the clams in my meal. Germs normally found in the clam proliferated after the clam's death and the clam "went bad," as we say, at a point after its demise. As the germs multiplied, they released toxins so that when I swallowed them they were crossing the line between unpalatability and poisonousness. The process is quite different from the transmission of clam-related hepatitis. In this case the clam can be quite alive and healthy and remain so until it is part of our meal. The hepatitis clam, however, is harvested from waters contaminated with sewage carrying a virus that is a harmless part of the clam's diet (harmless to the clam, that is). Hepatitis is not food poisoning, but the transmission of a virus.

When we speak of food poisoning, the toxicity is always caused by germs, either ones that infect us or ones that leave their toxins in the food we have consumed. Such is the case of ptomaine poisoning, as when staph germs shed from a food handler and find their way into the mayonnaise at the church picnic. The warmth of a summer afternoon is all the staph need to thrive in the mayonnaise, covertly spoiling it and, a few hours after the picnic, putting the parishioners on their knees praying for sufficient intervals between alternating obligations to sit or kneel. Human experience with the bad things that germs can do is as long as human experience itself, so the liver does not need lessons in ferreting out ptomaine and other toxins that may escape detection before food is swallowed. Most of the time when food spoils it is because of germs—bacteria and molds—that are present on or in the food when it is fresh and proliferate slowly even in the refrigerator unless the food has been treated to prevent or retard spoilage. The common ways to keep the germs down are heat sterilization and canning, complete drying, or the addition of enough sugar, salt or acid to poison any germs present and discourage their overgrowth. There is however, another way for food to go bad. It has to do with bad fat. The taste buds protect us from rancid fats. Rancid fat is not likely to get past the taste buds. The palate is otherwise not helpful in protecting us from eating fats that are bad or in selecting fats that are good in ways that have nothing to do with rancidity. Once fat is metabolized and becomes part of the body, we need to be able to keep it from going rancid in the body.

# CHAPTER 8

# Fat Is Not Just to Hold Your Pants Up

## THE IMPORTANCE OF ESSENTIAL OILS

ANDREA WAS A NINE-YEAR-OLD GIRL who was referred to me by a psychologist after she and her family had engaged in two years of therapy for her unpredictable outbursts of rage. She also had difficulty concentrating, was spacy, had mild fine motor clumsiness and adequate school performance. She had always been healthy although she had a history of cradle cap as an infant and, as her mother reported in her questionnaire, in the past Andrea had had a history of "chicken skin" on the backs of her upper arms. As I went through the questionnaire with Andrea and her mother I could not find any other diagnostic clues to Andrea's problems. When I then came to her physical exam I discovered that her mother forgot to mention that Andrea had been consulting a dermatologist for two years for a completely different problem. Her feet were constantly painful, dry and cracked. The skin was shiny in certain places and in others it was thick and callused with deep painful fissures that sometimes would bleed. She wore white cotton socks to bed and found some relief from steroid creams. The rest of Andrea's skin was smooth and lustrous, as was her hair. There was nothing wrong with her nails.

Although severe and very localized, Andrea's foot condition was in the spectrum of problems I see in children and adults who need more essential oils in their diets. In such cases there is an imbalance of oils, with too many "stiff" oils and too few "flexible" oils. These individuals need an oil change. If I saw Andrea today I might not feel the need to do a test of her oils. I would be more confident that her physical signs clearly indicated the need for essential oils. Fifteen years ago when I was treating Andrea, I was just beginning to understand[9] the full scope of the oil problem and a lab test was helpful in making my case for treatment. It showed that Andrea was deficient in the omega-3 fats, a major component of flaxseed oil. I suggested to her mother that she take a tablespoon of flaxseed oil daily. Within a couple of weeks, her feet became completely normal. Her outbursts of rage stopped within a month.

Here are a few more stories to give you an idea of the scope of the problem of insufficient fatty acids before I explain how it all works. Sandra Tiepolo was the sister of a long-standing patient who called me in distress to report that Sandra had a cancerous lesion discovered at the opening of her vagina. Her doctor was considering very extensive surgery that would have left Sandra crippled as far as sex and reproduction were concerned. The lesion was indeed a very scary-looking, cancerous one. In addition, Sandra had severe dandruff, dry skin, brittle fingernails, chicken skin on the backs of her arms and alligator skin on her legs. She was a catalogue of the physical signs of omega-3 fatty acid deficiency. I suggested that Sandra begin to replenish her oils while watching her lesion very closely and deferring surgery as long as some immediate improvement was noted. She took a tablespoon or two of flaxseed oil daily. Within days her dandruff began to clear, as did the other signs of fatty acid deficiency. Within a couple of weeks her cancerous lesion began to regress, and we watched it disappear over the ensuing 13 months. The happy ending is that Sandra subsequently married and had a daughter who is a teenager now.

Sarah was the sister of a medical student who did a clerkship with me. After seeing patients with me, my student asked her sister to come and visit so that I could look at the rash on her chest and hear her story of depression and failure to menstruate for the previous two years. She had an unusual rash on her chest that was a slightly raised, linear, pink to yellow color with faintly waxy texture and it had waxed and waned for two years. I hadn't seen anything exactly like it on someone's chest before nor have I since then. If it had been on Sarah's face at the edge of her hair line I would have called it seborrhea. Seborrhea, dandruff, scalp "itch-bumps" and mild psoriasis are all skin problems in which there is a local production of too much skin material which results in dandruff flakes and the crusting of other lesions. I saw her rash within this spectrum. I consider that spectrum a reliable sign that a person needs more omega-3 oils. I suggested that Sarah take a tablespoon of flaxseed oil daily and said that I was quite sure that it would take care of her rash as well as the rest of her problems. During the next month her skin cleared beautifully, her periods resumed and her mood became normal.

Signs of fatty acid problems—basically omega-3 oil deficiency— are among the most reliable among the subtle findings in the nutritional assessment of patients. For reasons I will explain in a moment these signs can be found in a large proportion of "normal" people as well as in those with a wide variety of health problems. Fatty acid chemistry is deep, and the way its abnormalities are reflected on the surface and in the symptoms of individuals can be quite varied. The clues that can be observed on the skin, however, fall into a spectrum in which a theme of dryness is manifested in different ways. They are:

1. Cracking finger tips—worse in winter.
2. Patchy dullness of the skin, especially on the face, with a subtle patchy variation in the color of the skin.
3. Mixed oily and dry skin which, in cosmetic advertisements, is sometimes called combination skin.
4. Chicken skin *(phrynoderma, hyperkeratosis follicularis)*, which constitutes small, rough bumps on the back of the arms.

5. Alligator skin, usually on the lower legs, which develop an irregular quilted appearance with dry patches.
6. Stiff, dry, unmanageable, brittle hair.
7. Seborrhea, cradle cap, dandruff, hair loss.
8. Soft fingernails or brittle fingernails which fray with horizontal splitting.

These findings usually respond dramatically when a person takes a supplement of omega-3 oils. Associated symptoms, sometimes including severe problems such as the ones I have described above, often melt away as the skin signs do. The variety of problems that respond to omega-3 fatty acid supplementation crosses all the boundaries between systems, specialties and diseases. Most people who have skin signs of fatty acid problems use various kinds of lotions, oils, shampoos, conditioners and cosmetics to cover their problems, often to no avail.

## WHY OILS CAN HEAL OR HARM

How can it be that not eating, or eating certain oils could make such a difference in people's health? The subject is very thoroughly covered in several good books, so I will only give you a summary and my particular viewpoint here. The toxicity of bad oils and the benefits of good oils represent a very different kind of problem in detoxification from all the others I describe in this book. The toxicity is far from poisoning in the sense of what happened to the ambassador's daughter and yet I believe it is the most common kind of poisoning that a practicing physician can find in his or her patients today.

Most of us have been taught to think of fat as basically dangerous, something to be avoided for the sake of one's health. In my medical training the chemistry of lipids, a more technical term for fats, received little attention. No other factor in nutrition has gone from such a lowly to such an exalted position as my understanding of the importance of oils to health. Fats and oils have three quite different roles in the body, two of which account for the major shift in my appreciation of the subject. The same two roles of fatty acids, as certain lipids are known, explain their enormous significance to health as exemplified in the cases I just described. After a brief description of each role of fatty acids, I will highlight a few key details.

1. The first role of fat is to hold up your pants, or otherwise provide the bulges and curves that belong to a well-rounded person. The fats and oils in your diet that become your body fat are an efficient form of stored energy. It is basically the only way the body has to store fuel that can carry you several hours beyond your last meal. Unlike plants, human beings do not have any way to store large amounts of carbohydrates to serve as stable reservoirs of energy. However, the liver does store some carbohydrate as glycogen that provides some energy during the initial day of a fast or during prolonged exercise. We can store fats, which some plants do as well. Nuts and seeds are the best example of plant stores of fat.

2. The second role of fat in your body is to make waterproof membranes. In this case I am not referring to membranes such as the surface of an organ or the mucous membranes, lining the inner passageways of your body. I am referring to cell membranes. Your body is made of cells, which are units of life. Life goes on only in the watery environment inside cells, whose water has a special composition quite different from the water outside of cells, whether that be seawater in the case of single cell organisms, fresh water or the water of your blood or in the spaces between the cells of complex organisms. Every cell is enclosed in a membrane that provides the waterproofing that enables it to separate its inside water from the water of its surroundings. The cell membrane is made of an uninterrupted fabric made of oil molecules.

3. The third role of oil molecules in your body is to become hormones. Usually, when you hear the word "hormone," you think of substances such as thyroid hormone or estrogen, testosterone, cortisol and other "steroid" hormones. Another category of hormones is less familiar to most people, partly because these, the prostanoid hormones, were discovered more recently (in the 1960s) and because they do not have an affiliation with a particular organ. Moreover, shortages of these hormones produce symptoms that do not fit as

neatly into the picture of a disease as do shortages of the other well-known hormones. Prostanoid hormones are made exclusively from fatty acids.

Keep these three roles of fatty acids—energy storage, water-proofing cell membranes and hormone synthesis—in mind as we explore the ways fatty acids can be toxic or beneficial.

## You *Are* What You Eat

Our palate for oils is blunt. I am sure that there are chefs and gour-mets who can taste test olive oil and determine its provenance as can an experienced oenologist tell the year and vineyard of a particular wine. When it comes to oils, however, most of us can barely distin-guish between samples of mineral oil, olive oil, safflower oil, flax-seed oil and motor oil when they are presented to be sniffed, touched and (except for the motor oil) tasted. I have experimented with audi-ences to demonstrate that we tend toward taste blindness when at-tempting to distinguish among the various oils. This is the reason the concept of "vegetable oil" or "salad oil" was readily accepted among Americans in the 1950s when corn and other oils came onto a market which previously offered only olive oil, lard, butter and margarine. Even families with a solid tradition of using culinary olive oil could be persuaded to switch to various mongrel oils sold in the supermarket. Such oils, extracted from various plant seeds by means of hot steel rollers and a process that involves dissolving and recovering the oils from a solvent similar to dry cleaning fluid, were sold with the assumption that this clear, pure-appearing stuff was what we consumers wished to (or could be made to wish to) eat. The oils were also marketed with an eye to shelf life, so that a bottle of vegetable oil that languished on the shelf of the general store would not go bad over a period of months. Some of the oils that could be squeezed and dissolved out of, say, a corn kernel, are quite suscepti-ble to spoilage while others are very stable, so that removing the vulnerable fraction of the oil resulted in a product of remarkable stability. The problem is that the oils that were removed are nutri-tionally valuable, while the ones that remain are nutritionally undesirable or even toxic. Still, these altered oils may taste just fine. They are toxic not because they are rancid but because they have been altered to lengthen their shelf life. The result is a man-made oil that provides us with molecules we do not need and which deprives us of those we do need. Our taste buds are hopeless at giving us the slightest clue that this has happened.

Toxic oils are probably the most important issue in human health in our time, but the effects of their toxicity are quite different from those presented by my clam experience, Hillary's red dye experience, the ambassador's daughter's tick, or Luke's estrogen overload. All you need to understand oils and fats derives from three simple sets of facts.

### 1. Whatever fats you eat become your fat.

I have just explained that our sense of taste can't discriminate between different kinds of oils and fats. They are so interchangeable as to be listed on labels of prepared foods as "one or the other of the following." The manufacturer is then free to use whatever source of shortening is currently most available or cheapest on the market. Whatever fats you eat become *your* fat. Contrary to the points I made in the previous chapter, dietary fats enter the fat stores and cell membranes without being altered. If you eat chicken fat, your fat reflects the fatty acid composition of the chicken. If you were to eat only fat from olive oil, then your body's fat composition would reveal the distinctive proportions of the main fatty acids in olives. Unlike proteins and carbohydrates, dietary fatty acids come into the body by a very direct path and are neither identified nor, for the most part, disassembled and reassembled. On the other hand, the protein of your body is distinctively yours: if you eat cow's muscle or drink cow's milk your muscle and your secretions still retain your own distinctive human composition. The same is true for carbohydrates. Not so with fat.

The body is capable of making all kinds of fatty molecules that are similar to the ones in your diet (except for two), but usually, it does not bother to do so; it uses the fat molecules (fatty acids) that you have eaten. After you swallow your food, the fats and oils are separated from the carbohydrate and protein as they pass through the upper part of the intestine. The carbohydrate, which is broken down into sugars, and the protein, which is broken down into amino acids, pass into the liver where they can be monitored for any properties that are foreign to your nature and altered accordingly. The fatty acids in the fat you eat go by an entirely different route directly from the digestive tract into the bloodstream. This path consists of a vessel which delivers all the fats and oils of your meal directly to a large blood vessel at the base of the neck just below the collar bone. The whole concept of digestion is therefore different as far as fats are concerned as compared with carbohydrate and protein. In the case of fats, their digestion is nondestructive and intended only to convert the fats and oils into tiny droplets that can float into the blood as milk fats are suspended in whole fresh milk before homogenization.

*2. The only two fats you cannot make, but have to get from food, are the raw materials for making a whole family of important hormones.*

This is one of the most important scientific facts I have learned since before college when Mr. Mayo-Smith began to teach me biology beginning with the notion that there are a few pivotal facts that give leverage to thinking. To recap: when it comes to fat, you are what you eat. Although the body has the capacity to make fat molecules on its own (for example, from sugar), it generally does not do so. However, there are two essential fatty acids that the body cannot make. The pivotal fact here is that these two fatty acid molecules are the exclusive raw materials for making *all* of the prostanoid hormones. Let me put it another way: the body has a constant need to synthesize, manufacture, create, build an assortment of substances called prostanoid hormones, the main vehicles for communication from cell to cell in the body. Unlike steroid hormones that are synthesized in special glands (adrenals, ovaries, testicles) or thyroid hormones which come exclusively from the thyroid gland, the prostanoid hormones are made by just about every cell in the body. Steroid and thyroid hormones are examples of long-distance message carriers originating in organs that are remote from the tissues throughout the body where their message is targeted. Prostanoid hormones are more involved with short-distance message carrying, and there is no special organ in the body that has the exclusive job of producing them. A whole orchestra of prostanoid hormones are in constant production. Their combined effect is like music that cells play to their neighbors to keep their mutual efforts harmonized. All of the instruments of this music are made out of the two kinds of fat molecule that have to be eaten regularly to supply the necessary raw materials. It seems extraordinary to me that Mother Nature made us entirely dependent on our diet to supply these two molecules when we have a full capacity to produce at least a couple of dozen other molecules that differ from them in what appear to be only minor details.

The names of the two essential fatty acids are linoleic acid and alpha-linolenic acid. Omega-3 fatty acids are the family of fatty acids we make from alpha-linolenic acid. When the manufacturers of vegetable oil developed methods for squeezing various seeds to extract their oils, and various kinds of "salad" or "cooking" oils hit the market in the 1950s, the oils were able to survive on grocery shelves for months without becoming rancid because the manufacturers removed the alpha-linolenic acid, the oil that has the greatest tendency to rancidity. At the time, no one knew that linoleic acid and alpha-linolenic acid had crucial roles as the exclusive precursors of all of the prostanoid hormones. Prostanoid hormones would not be discovered, nor their chemistry unraveled, until more than a decade later.

*3. All of the cell membranes of the body are made of fatty acids. Cell membranes need to be flexible to function. The two fatty acids we cannot make are the flexible ones.*

Their unique role in prostanoid hormone chemistry would be enough to place the role of fatty acids in hormone production among the top few items in my biochemical knowledge. However, the use of fatty acids for making cell membranes is a corollary fact that puts it at the very top. Life goes on in cells, not in the spaces in between. In order for all the cells (100,000,000,000,000 or $10^{13}$ of them) to function optimally, they must be able to communicate with each other. Prostanoid hormones are one of the most important means for such communication. Each individual cell must be open to such communication while at the same time it must be closed off from the water that surrounds it. The fabric of their waterproof membranes is a velvet made of fatty acids forming the nap. Each tiny strand that forms the surface of the velvet is a fatty acid, a long skinny molecule standing on its end amidst millions of others in all directions, each nested against the other like stacked spoons. One layer of fatty acid velvet faces inward to the inside of the cell and another faces outward, and the whole arrangement owes its most important property (being waterproof) to the fact that oil and water do not mix. There is water inside the membrane and water outside the membrane but the membrane itself does not get wet.

Unlike the cells of plants and fungi, the cell membrane is not a wall. It is a delicate diaphanous fabric with a flexibility more like silk than velvet. It must be so in order to accommodate one of the main functions of the membrane: communication. That is, it must be able to form various kinds of pockets in which protein and carbohydrate molecules float in the fat to be receptor sites for messenger molecules coming from other cells. For the cell membrane to be flexible it must be made of flexible oils. Which are the most flexible oils? You guessed it: linoleic acid and, especially, alpha-linolenic acid. Alpha-linolenic acid owes its flexibility to the same property that makes it vulnerable to giving up electrons and thus becoming oxidized or rancid; it is very unsaturated. Alpha-linolenic acid is the queen of the polyunsaturated fatty acids and the mother of the omega-3 family of fatty acids.

Essentially, all of the business of the body is conducted within membranes. Those that surround the cell, however important, are part of a much larger system of membranes inside each cell that support the activities of cellular life. If you were to take the measure of the surface membrane of each cell and multiply it by the number of cells in the body, the total surface area would be as large as a tennis court or two. As for the total surface area of all the membranes inside the cells, this would be about the size of 10 football fields. It takes a lot of flexible fatty acids to keep these membranes flexible; this is crucial because the stiffer they are, the less well they work.

How does this flexibility—or lack thereof—manifest itself in your health? The stiff and weakening changes in hair, skin and nails are easy to see in terms of the effects of a lack of fatty acids that have to do with flexibility. The changes that result in hormonal imbalances and cellular damage leading to cancer, heart disease and other major problems are more difficult to visualize. Moreover, the chain of cause and effect is more complex than, say, the way a tick toxin or an egg allergy can make you sick. The complexity of understanding cause and effect increases as you are asked to make a distinction between bad fats and good fats. Simply put, the "good" fats are the thin ones that make flexible cell membranes and prostanoid hormones. The "bad" ones are the stiff ones, the altered oils from which the good fatty acids have been removed.

Fat can harm the body in three ways, two of which you cannot taste. The third, rancidity, tastes so unpleasant that your taste buds know how to protect you. Let's begin with the first two.

When vegetable oils are extracted and processed from seeds and nuts, two kinds of damage occur to their fatty acid molecules. The damage is related to two of the ways fat can "go bad." In the first way, the pressure and heat of the extracting process causes some of the molecules to undergo rotation at one of their "joints," where two carbon atoms have a double connection with each other. As a result, the molecules change shape. The curve that normally occurs at each double connection becomes reversed so that the molecule is straightened. Recall that in the cell membrane the molecules are nested together like stacked spoons. Straightened ones lose their capacity to fit together in the velvet of the cell membranes. The transformation into an unnatural, straightened fatty acid is one which technical terminology designates as a "trans" configuration. Except for those that are cold-pressed, processed oils tend to have more or less trans fatty acids which stiffen the cell membranes. They are also unsuited for use as raw materials for making prostanoid hormones.

Margarine tends to have an especially high percentage of trans fatty acids. Margarine, however, is especially toxic for other reasons. Its oils have been intentionally altered and straightened by another process called hydrogenation. Hydrogenation consists of bubbling hydrogen through an oil under conditions in which hydrogen joins fatty acid molecules at the double connections between carbon atoms. The addition of the hydrogen atoms can occur only if half of the double connection is converted for hydrogen holding. Once the new hydrogen is added at these points, the double connections are lost as the fatty acid becomes more saturated with respect to hydrogen. The end result is an oil that has changed from thin and flexible to thick and stiff. The resulting thick and stiff oil resembles fats and oils that are naturally thick and stiff, such as one finds in fattened animals and in naturally saturated oils. Thick and stiff oils are toxic in that they cause an unwelcome rigidity in cell membranes and do not provide suitable raw materials for making hormones. The symptoms, physical signs of dry skin or hair and the medical problems of the patients I described earlier can all be understood in terms of the effects of too many altered (trans or stiffened) fatty acids and an insufficiency of good, flexible oils.

The reason that flaxseed oil is especially medicinal for individuals who require an oil change is that it has an exceptional concentration (about 40 percent) of the thinnest, most flexible alpha-linolenic oil of all seeds and nuts. The next closest in concentration are walnuts and rapeseed, the source of canola oil. Each of these oils has about one-fourth the concentration of flaxseed oil. Flaxseed oil is a traditional food oil in parts of Eastern Europe such as the Ukraine. Its plant source is used for making linen cloth, and its small pointed brown seeds yield their oils when pressed by old-fashioned methods available before the modern hot steel rollers used so widely today. Antioxidants are abundant in oils that are freshly pressed by old-fashioned methods that yield a turbid product that would seem dirty looking to the eye of consumers accustomed to transparent "pure" oils. The apparent "impurities" in these oils are actually parts of the crushed seed that contain the antioxidants that permit seeds to stay fresh during prolonged storage. Similarly these antioxidants, such as vitamin E, protect the unrefined oil when stored or heated in ways that are not recommended for purified oils. Family members who grew up on old-fashioned flaxseed oil tell me that it would stay fresh all year without refrigeration and that its taste was much more agreeable than the flaxseed oils that are currently available in the United States. Flaxseed, or linseed, oil was used in Eastern European homes as the principal edible oil for cooking. It was also used medicinally for treating burns where its effectiveness may be due to its generous content of antioxidants. Its effectiveness in treating a wide variety of skin, hair and nail problems and much deeper underlying medical disorders is owed to its capacity to restore flexibility to cell membranes and replenish the supply of raw materials for prostaglandin hormone synthesis.

The most concise way of describing the superficial effects of restoring the body's supply of alpha-linolenic acid is to say that it gives luster. When we are in good health, we show a glow of health about us. Such a glow is easily recognized but difficult to describe except that it has to do with the emission or reflection of light. It is no coincidence that flaxseed oil is the unique vehicle for oil paint pigments where it imparts a luster to paintings that cannot be duplicated by another oil. When a painter runs out of linseed oil, he or she does not accept substitution with olive, corn or coconut oil. Neither should you. And, when your skin gets dull and dry, you should consider whether your oil needs changing before you reach for a cream, lotion, oil or cosmetic to cover up the problem.

Are there tests to measure what you are missing? Serious alterations in the kinds of fatty acids in your blood and cell membranes can be detected by ordinary quantitative tests for fatty acids. Even so, such tests are available only at special laboratories.[10] Early stages of fatty acid deficiency are common in North Americans who consume mostly altered or saturated fats. The analysis of blood to detect these abnormalities is the special interest of Dr. Eduardo Siguel, who has developed the technology to measure early changes in the proportions of good and bad fatty acids including Mead acid, which the body starts to make for use in cell membranes when it runs out of alpha-linolenic acid. Mead acid lacks the proper shape and flexibility of the real thing. However, it is all the body can do in a pinch and it is one of the keys to Dr. Siguel's method for fatty acid deficiency determination.[11] Dr. Siguel's book[12] provides a comprehensive review of the subject, and several of his recent papers describe essential fatty acid deficiency as the key to coronary artery disease,[13] a common complication of digestive disorders,[14] and one of the most misunderstood aspects of various prevailing recommendations concerning a healthy diet.[15-18]

I have described three basic facts about oils: 1. You are what you eat, 2. Good oils provide for the flexibility of cell membranes and 3. They are the raw materials for making the prostanoid hormones. I have discussed two of the three ways that dietary fats can be toxic: when they are misshapen or when they are stiff. Rancidity, the remaining way that fats can be toxic, can happen before or after they enter your body. Our taste buds (actually our sense of smell) are so sensitive to rancid changes in oils and fats that we are quite well protected from consuming oils that have gone bad in this way. The same damage that constitutes rancidity can happen after fatty acid molecules have reached their destination in our bodies. It is worth understanding the details of what happens to fatty acids when they become rancid, because once you have grasped that process you will be able to understand the most globally toxic force affecting *all* of the molecules of the body, the enemy of youth, the ally of all diseases, and the fundamental mechanism of all injury, deterioration, aging and death: oxidation.

If oils are extracted in the old-fashioned way, without heat or chemicals, they retain many of the protective substances that keep them from going bad. Only when oils are filtered and refined to remove these protective substances and make them clear do they become subject to oxidation or what we know as rancidity. So far I have referred to the toxic properties of fats in terms of their texture—stiff or flexible. Because the texture of the fats in your body is completely dependent on the flexibility of the fats in your diet, it makes sense to favor flexible oils over stiff oils. Your palate may be quite blind to the different viscosity, saturation, stiffness or omega factor of various oils but it is relatively acute when it comes to rancidity. So you may say, "What is the problem? I don't eat any rancid oils." Indeed, you have a built-in capacity to taste rancidity when it is present at a very dilute concentration in any oil that you eat. You may be quite blind to the big difference between mineral oil and vegetable oil but you have an acute sense of the difference between a fresh oil and one that has just begun to turn. However, as far as the body is concerned, rancidity's ill effect really occurs after you eat damaged oils (which may taste perfectly fine) and they become part of cell membranes. Thus it is essential to good health not to allow the body's oils to become rancid.

The following illustrative skit will provide a metaphor for understanding not only what happens when fats become oxidized or rancid, but also the series of events that protect fats and all of our other living molecules from undergoing the same damage. These events are important to understanding oxidation and antioxidants, which are as important as they are complex. The complexity of antioxidants may be easier for you to keep in mind if you use your visual memory; hence the following short play is offered for you to envision.

The first character is the Juggler, who represents a fatty acid molecule with its electrons in the air. The Juggler could, however, be any molecule in the body including DNA. The second character is the Rogue, who represents any kind of oxidative stress. The third is Ascorbia, the lady in white, playing the role of vitamin C. Other players will appear as the scene unfolds.

Imagine the Juggler in a crowd of tourists. He is magnificent, able to keep seven objects in the air, a swarm of sparkling items that shine like the sequins of his costume. It almost seems as if he is casting parts of his very self into the air as the rhythmic simplicity of his juggling captivates us and compels us to give him room in the crowd. Now there is a disruption at the edge of the onlookers as a busybody emerges and violates the space around the Juggler. It is the greedy young Rogue charging the Juggler and shouting, "I want one, I want one." Enter Ascorbia, dressed in white, stepping from the crowd to intervene just as the Juggler begins to feel the pull of the Rogue's approach. "Don't take his," she cries, "take mine," and she holds out a sparkling article which disappears in the grasp of the Rogue. The entertainment continues as the crowd offers grateful glances to Ascorbia who, however, is bereft of her sparkling article and looking sad until Bio Flavinoid, her companion dressed in yellow, offers her one just like it. She is soothed, but now Bio Flavinoid slips from the crowd with an air of dejection that is immediately broken by the bounding presence of a large golden retriever named Carrots, who lays a shimmering sphere at the feet of Bio Flavinoid and then runs off. If we were to follow Carrots, we would see her head straight for an old man named V. E. Shute with baggy pants and pockets glowing with replacements for the sparkling objects. Mr. Shute is visited regularly and replenished by a princely figure, Regie or reduced glutathione(RG), whom we will describe more fully in chapter 9.

If the sparkling objects are electrons, then the Juggler, the members of the crowd, the lady, her companion, the dog and the old man are all molecules. Let's replace the Juggler with a fatty acid molecule. The unruly rogue could be any of several kinds of oxidative stress that have a common greed for electrons. Atmospheric oxygen is the most abundant of such electron-hungry substances. We use it to enable us to take electrons from the sugar and fat molecules we use for fuel. The disassembly of our fuel molecules is accomplished by the removal of their electrons. The need for oxygen to do this, however, threatens us with the prospect that the molecules we wish to keep intact are subject to oxygen's burning influence. Suffice it to say that it is oxygen and all related oxidative stresses that put our molecules at risk of losing an electron. Such a loss is a necessary part of all chemistry in which molecules participate voluntarily. All chemistry has to do with the sharing, gaining or losing of electrons from one atom or molecule (a collection of atoms whose electrons swarm together).

The involuntary or inadvertent loss of electrons from molecules whose integrity is important to the structure of our cell membranes, DNA, the skin or the clear substances in the eye results in damage or disease. The oxidative stress may be physical trauma, chemical exposure, the wear and tear of aging, or a burn which is oxidation in its most extreme form.

The fire from a candle flame aptly illustrates oxidation in which the electrons of the candle wax are ripped off by oxygen in the atmosphere with the resulting, self-perpetuating release of light and heat. If a fatty acid molecule gets its electron ripped off by oxygen in the air, it is damaged. If the fatty acid molecule is a pat of butter or olive oil, we call the damage "rancidity." If the fatty acid molecule is nested among millions of others in the velvety pile of our cell membranes, we call the damage "oxidative damage" or "peroxidation."

If one cell membrane fatty acid molecule loses its electron, its neighbors feel the suction of the loss and a collective destabilization occurs so that whole area of the membrane becomes more easily oxidized and thus damaged, altered, misshapen and stiffened.

Enter vitamin C, an antioxidant whose companion, the bioflavinoids, aid in the transfer of a replacement electron. Beta-carotene is a necessary bridge in the transfer of a new electron from vitamin E, which is replenished in turn by glutathione. In the end the replacements are supplied by a nutrient-rich diet. However, the path from dietary intake to antioxidant protection through the generosity of vitamin C is dependent on an inflexible sequence that is very much like a bucket brigade and it quenches a problem that is very much like a fire.

Another firefighter's instrument, a ladder, is an even better image than a bucket brigade for understanding antioxidants. It is an especially good metaphor to underline the flaws in various research efforts that cast doubt on the value or safety of particular antioxidants. A recent study[19] of vitamin E and beta-carotene in heavy smokers in Finland suggested that beta-carotene might be dangerous because of its statistical association with a higher incidence of lung cancer in men who took supplements of beta-carotene as part of a long-term experiment studying the effects of vitamin E and/or beta-carotene supplementation. The antioxidant brigade is like a ladder: it depends on the presence of all of the rungs for its safe operation. Modern scientific thinking favors experiments in which a very limited number of variables are studied while all the other circumstances are controlled. That approach translates into selecting a single drug, nutrient or other intervention to be studied, avoiding the confusion that would result from the introduction of several variables at once.

The same question comes up every day in my practice. After taking a history and doing tests that indicate a lack of certain nutrients and/or the presence of certain allergens or toxins, I suggest that my patient undertake several remedial steps at once. These may also include advice to exercise, learn diaphragmatic breathing, meditate or verbalize strong feelings such as anger or grief. "But how will we know what is working?" asks an occasional patient. "If you get better, you may be quite confused. It is preferable to be confused and better than to be so selective that progress may be impossible. Remember that if you are sitting on two tacks and you remove just one, you will not feel 50 percent better. Chronic illness is multifactorial. It is downright negligent to focus so exclusively on a single treatment that you fail to address the whole picture.

What about the Finnish smokers? The researchers who carried out the experiment followed an understandable, but in this case, inappropriate, instinct to be selective. They chose to study only one or two antioxidants that function as members of a team of many. One, beta-carotene, becomes toxic itself if it cannot become replenished by vitamin E, which in turn, runs short if sufficient supplies of riboflavin (vitamin $B_2$) are not available. It is as if a study were designed to validate that ladders are useful tools for firefighters to climb to put out a fire by breaking the ladder down to its components and testing each one individually. Such a study would prove that individual ladder rungs are not only useless, but potentially dangerous. The Finnish smokers experiment was conducted with scientific precision. Its flaw was a fundamental ignorance of antioxidant chemistry. Antioxidants do not work alone.

Fat is arguably the most important material in the body. It is responsible for the packaging of every cell, the membranous support for most cellular activity and the raw material for making the hormones that communicate between cells. As this picture has emerged over the past 30 years, it was a revelation to me. When I went to medical school the chemistry of fat was glossed over as dull and unimportant. It is even more surprising to me that the cholesterol frenzy of recent years has taken precedence over the significance of good fatty acids. By good fatty acids I mean not only alpha-linolenic and linoleic acids, but the avoidance of factors that introduce stiffness and flaws into the fabric of our fatty membrane acreage. Eating stiff (saturated) or altered (trans, hydrogenated) fats is a problem because the palate is absolutely no help in protecting us from the toxicity of these molecules. I reemphasize that rancid fats are a problem not because we tend to eat so much of them, but because oxidation threatens our fatty acid molecules after they are eaten and have already taken up their proper place in our membranes. As we will

explore presently, oxidative damage is a threat to nearly all molecules in our body, but the threat to fatty acids has a special twist.
Remember that when they are membrane molecules, fatty acid "jugglers" are not alone in a crowd but are members of a continuous
formation of jugglers packed together like a marching band in tight
formation. Oxidative damage affects them more than other molecules in the body because of the domino effect that occurs when one
of their fatty acids becomes oxidized.

There is a big molecule, superoxide dismutase, that can actually
grab and subdue oxidative stress before vitamin C comes to the
rescue. For the most part, however, the protection of our fatty acid
membranes and other important molecules is a quintessentially co-
operative enterprise in which hundreds of molecules that are not
ordinarily considered antioxidants can lend a hand (or an electron)
when the need arises. The failure of antioxidant protection yields a
toxic effect on molecules of all kinds. The molecules that are the
most precious jewels of our chemistry are the DNA which carry the
instructions that maintain our identity in each of the cells as well as
our ancestral identity.

# CHAPTER 9

# DNA:
# The Family Jewels

I AM NOT SURE when I first heard gonads referred to as "the family jewels;" it was probably during recess in the fourth grade when contact sports increased the risk of gonadal injury at a time when my schoolmates and I experienced the dawning of interest in reproductive physiology. I understood the value of those jewels in terms of avoiding the pain that might come from a misdirected kick or elbow, or a fall onto a fence or the bar that distinguished my bike as a boy's bike with its special peril for boys' gonads. I misunderstood a number of details concerning the reproductive value of the jewelry and, even when I got the basic facts straight, I still did not understand that I was the protector of the genetic material of a family that extended immeasurably above me to my ancestors and might extend continuously below me to those whose ancestor I would someday be. I certainly did not understand that oxidative stress was a greater threat than the crossbar on my bicycle to my DNA (genes, chromosomes, genetic endowment).

DNA or deoxyribonucleic acid is inherently less susceptible to oxidation than the very unsaturated fatty acids of my cell membranes. The latter have electrons that are particularly susceptible to being grabbed by any other molecule, such as oxygen, that has a hunger for them. Fatty acids are crucial to the structure of cells and serve as raw material for making hormones, but DNA is the bearer of information from the past to the future. If the cell membrane becomes damaged, the cell's function may suffer. If DNA becomes damaged, the misinformation that results may engender more serious and lasting consequences: for you, if it is in any cell of your body; or for your offspring, if it is in one of the few eggs or sperms that you will use to make a family. The integrity of your DNA is so important that you have a repair mechanism to fix DNA molecules in any cell of your body. If the messages of the previous chapter were, "Keep your membranes flexible" or "Hang on to your electrons," then the moral of this one is, "Maintain your DNA."

Meet SAM. SAM is a molecule with a long name, s-adenosyl-methionine, so we call it SAM for short. It is a relatively small molecule, a few times bigger than a fatty acid, and you wouldn't even notice it next to a DNA molecule which is made up of thousands of units, each of which is about SAM's size. SAM has an exclusive franchise, a distributorship. SAM has cornered the market for delivering the most fundamental material needed for making and repairing molecules all over your biochemistry: single carbon atoms in the form of methyl groups, which we can call methyl. There is no molecule in your body that is not based on carbon atoms. Carbohydrate, fat, protein, hormones, neurotransmitters and all of the other hundred thousand different kinds of molecules that make up your body are all based on the stringing together of carbon atoms, which in turn may connect with oxygens, hydrogens, nitrogens, sulfur, phosphorus and so on. The fundamental structural unit, a carbon atom, is so ubiquitous and so apparently available that it seems odd that there is a need for special arrangements to have it delivered to wherever it is needed for new construction or repair and it seems even more odd that there should be just one guy with the whole franchise. I would have thought that such special arrangements would be needed for nitrogen. It is needed for the synthesis of all sorts of important molecules—amino acids, proteins and nucleic acids—and yet single nitrogens are moved easily from one molecule to another in a process of transamination. Indeed, the nitrogen we do obtain in our diet has to come more or less prepackaged in about a dozen essential amino acids that serve as raw materials for important molecules (neurotransmitters, proteins). SAM, in fact, is made from one of these essential amino acids: methionine. SAM will re-enter my story after discovering a jewel thief at the shoe store.

I, the fourth grader, leave my boy's bike in the driveway and join my mother for a trip to two of my favorite stores: May's department store with escalators to ride, and Roentgen's shoe store, where you can look right at the bones of your feet in the X-ray machine.

I was delighted by the device that let me stand on a platform and watch a screen above it display my wiggling toe bones in action surrounded by the staccato images of the shoe nails and topped by the circles of eyelets for my laces. X-rays streamed through my feet and crashed into the phosphor on the fluoroscope screen where the particles of light (photons) were exchanged for some that I could see and that varied with the density encountered by the rays as they traversed my foot. This was really neat. My toes in action. Seeing the invisible. My mother would not let me linger long on the machine. No one else was waiting to use it, but one needed to set boundaries on how much fun to extract from the situation which did not have the natural limit of an ice cream cone. Propriety, not jeopardy, was the guideline. My mother did not conceive that there might be a danger to the family's DNA hanging in direct line of the X-rays.

The danger was that a high-energy photon would go crashing through my molecules and on the way it would knock off an electron which would need to be replaced, perhaps from a fatty acid in a cell membrane. Then either the cell membrane would suffer damage or vitamin C and all the other antioxidants would rescue the situation. As the X-ray photons streamed through my various parts, every molecule in my body was juggling its electrons. The potential for damage depended not only on the local supply of antioxidants but on the kind of cell and kind of molecule that might take the hit. As I changed my socks to try on a pair of sneakers, a few superficial skin cells would have been loosened to provide lunch for the dust mites that inhabited the carpet of the shoe store. If the fatty acid membranes of these cells had just been damaged by the passing X-rays, I would go free of harm. If some injury occurred to most of the parts of most of the cells of my body, the consequences would dissipate with the death of that cell in due course as the cell finished its allotted time.

If, however, the photon from the machine collided with a DNA molecule and knocked off an electron, this oxidative damage to the information stores of my body would threaten me in one of three ways unless the damage were to be repaired. One way could distort the information package presented by a dividing cell in any part of me so that its daughter cell, the daughter's daughters, and so on, could perpetuate the distortion, altering the function of a whole line of cells. Certain kinds of distorted information could lead to a line of cells that gave up their allegiance to me and set up an independent, cancerous existence as the ultimate effect of the hit from the machine in the shoe store. A second way could distort the information package of one of the permanent undividing cells of my brain or immune system and so pollute or diminish the irreplaceable small reservoir of the cells that form the basis of the self I was and would become. A third way could distort the information package of the family jewels. An alteration in the DNA of a sperm-producing cell, if not repaired, could harm the information entrusted to me by my ancestors and steal that legacy from my offspring.

I seem to have survived my trip to the shoe store. I continue to sense the presence of that same little boy in me still, and no maverick cells have caused any more of a threat than a few precancerous clusters on my bald head, where some tropical sun did the kind of damage that the shoe store X-rays appear to have failed to do. My daughters seem to carry a full set of ancestral genes. My DNA has remained functional despite countless oxidative attacks on the electrons of its doublestranded molecules. In some instances the lady in the white dress, her companion, the golden retriever and the rest of the oxidative protection team stepped in to prevent any harm. In other instances, the Rogue, more scientifically called "reactive oxygen species" or "free radicals," ran off with electrons, and sections of DNA lost their shape with a resulting loss of information as if pages were torn from a book. Enter SAM, the repair man with his supply of methyls to help replace broken parts in my DNA. Note that the broken part here is one that concerns information, not structure. The fatty acid velvet that make up the basic fabric of the cellular membranes of my body are important as components of these key structures. If membranes get damaged, the harm is limited to the cell in question and may be more or less important depending on whether the cell is transient or a part of my permanent cells. In either case the damage is not multiplied. If the damaged cell were to be one that does multiply (that is, divide), the defect would, if anything, be diluted in the process.

DNA, however, is a molecule that contains information. If it is damaged the harm will spread to future generations of the cell, which may be future generations of one's family if the cell is a sperm or an egg from which a child emerges. At the very least the damage will spread to the cells that arise from the afflicted cell unless the damage is repaired. An elaborate mechanism exists in the nucleus of each of your cells for the repair of DNA molecules that have been altered by oxidative damage. The crucial intermediary in that mechanism is folic acid, a B vitamin which has a major role in preventing cancer by supporting the synthesis of healthy DNA and the repair of damaged DNA.[20] The reason that we are so preoccupied by the toxic effects of radiation—from X-ray machines to sunlight—is that the damage it causes to DNA may be passed from cell to cell. Otherwise, it would not be worth the body's effort to nullify the effects of damage to DNA. As it stands the body's effort uses resources that come from the food we eat and the food we eat is often not sufficient even if we eat very well. The dose of folic acid required to assist in the repair of damaged DNA is well beyond the current RDA.

## THE IMPORTANCE OF FOLIC ACID

Some people with a special need for folic acid end up having babies with birth defects, others end up with heart disease, and still others with lung, esophageal, bowel or uterine cancers. Many people with any one of those problems got their problem from causes that have nothing to do with folic acid. Knowing the name and knowing the cause may be very different exercises.

If you came to me as a smoker, as a woman thinking about

starting a pregnancy, as a person with a history of colitis, as a woman with a repeatedly abnormal Pap smear, or as a person with a blood test indicating a high level of homocysteine, I would include the same steps as part of my recommendation: large doses of folic acid regardless of your diagnosis. In each case the folic acid has the same job working as SAM's agent in distributing methyls to DNA chemistry. Methylation is such an important part of chemistry that it deserves a status along with helping your molecules hang on to their electrons. We have already encountered the antioxidant team that prevents the theft of electrons. DNA is protected by the same antioxidant mechanisms, but its repair depends on an interconnected group of substances that have other additional important tasks worthy of your understanding. To illustrate this concept, I offer another complex metaphor, with my apologies for its old-fashioned cast of characters. The names and interrelationships of the substances I want to tell you about will probably enter your vocabulary in the next few years just as the names of several vitamins, minerals and amino acids may have done in the last few years. If I can give you some imagery to keep them straight you will have a head start. The biochemical task we are about to consider is the distribution of methyls, with particular attention to the repair of DNA.

Methionine is the queen of amino acids. There are 22 different amino acids in the royal family of nitrogen-bearing molecules, all but one of which* join together to form small aggregates of two to a dozen, known as peptides, or huge aggregates of thousands known as proteins. An elite group of amino acids have assignments as individuals** apart from contributing to the formation of peptides and proteins.

The queen of these few independent royal agents, Methionine, owes her monarchy to the special versatility of her triple endowment: 1) Methyls, single carbon units; 2) Sulfur, an element with

---

* Taurine. It functions as a free agent and does not make up a part of larger molecules. It can be used if consumed as such, but under ordinary circumstances it is made from methionine.

** For example, tyrosine is used for forming thyroid hormone as well as norepinephrine. Tryptophan is the raw material needed for making another neurotransmitter, serotonin.

important qualities of stickiness; and 3) Nitrogen, the defining ingredient of amino acids. Let us watch Methionine as she carries out her royal duties. She enters the courtroom carrying the methyl treasure. She receives a message that single carbon atoms are needed to repair the royal treasure house, where the genealogy and all the memories of the kingdom are preserved from generation to generation. She anticipates the (temporary) loss of her treasure and, unable to part with it and still maintain her identity, she dons a costume and becomes SAM. As SAM she can give up her methyl to folic acid, the subcontractor responsible for carrying the precious commodity for the repair of DNA. In so doing she is transformed to a mean, dangerous molecule that poses a great threat to the kingdom unless it is satisfied by being assigned to the kingdom's most valuable project (sanitation) or by being re-endowed with a methyl to recover its status. The dangerous molecule in question is Methionine's dark alter ego, Horrible Homocysteine. This molecule is a prime example of how toxic one's own chemistry can become without any influence from tick bites, germs, rancid oils or radiation. No matter what sort of toxic food you may eat, poisonous air you may breathe or contaminated water you may drink, you will have a hard time finding in your environment as mean a molecule as homocysteine. You have approximately one chance in 50 of being poisoned by your own homocysteine for the simple reason that you are not meeting your quirky needs for folic acid, vitamin B6 or vitamin $B_{12}$. The first warnings[21] of homocysteine's harmful habits came from a Harvard Medical School faculty member, Kilmer S. McCully, whose 1960 propositions have finally been confirmed 30 years after his initial reports were rejected by his colleagues.

In the first year of medical school we students heard stories about medical giants of the past who were hounded or even hung for their dissent from current views. I thought that our professors meant that such practices had been discontinued and that science had become open to the rapid acceptance of sound ideas and the fair treatment of their proponents. McCully is one of many people of the present generation whose treatment by his peers illustrates that science is not the objective realm of dispassionate weighers and measurers that it is cracked up to be. Even if it were, it might take years for any new idea to catch on while enduring the heat of scientific skepticism and suffering the necessary delays of publication, discussion and replication. The time it takes to get new ideas across is at least doubled by the workings of egos and personal conflicts that worm their way into any competitive activity.

When McCully fingered homocysteine he had a pretty good handle on how it might interact with oxidative stress to be the main cause of cardiovascular disease in many people. An up-to-date expansion and elaboration of his ideas by Stamler and Slivka[22] was brought to my attention by Jeffrey Bland who pointed out that this is one of the key articles in the current literature. It covers the interconnections of sulfur amino acid chemistry with many other activities in biochemistry. Here are the main points translated into the terms I have been using. If you understand them you will be able to grasp a number of related advances in chemistry that will influence your health over the next few years.

1. Methionine and its alter ego, homocysteine, have a relationship which exemplifies other situations in biochemistry in which a particularly helpful and healthful molecule is just one step away from being a particularly toxic one. The very properties that give value to a molecule (such as the combined close presence of sulfur-, nitrogen-, oxygen- and carbon-containing groups in methionine) can give rise to compounds that may be versatile and useful on the one hand or quite troublesome on the other.

2. As I will explain later, one of the chief ways our bodies quench the potential toxicity of hormones such as Luke's excess estrogen, as well as various neurotransmitters and all kinds of unwanted foreign molecules, is to stick on a sulfur-oxygen group called sulfate. In the case of the damage done by homocysteine, it appears that the main harm done to blood vessels and other tissues in the body is a misuse of sulfation so that healthy tissues are, in a distorted sense of the word, detoxified. As I mentioned previously and will describe more fully in chapter 15, detoxification involves adding sticky stuff to stinky molecules to render them more manageable. If you start sticking sulfates where they co-opt the desired adhesion between mole-

cules in healthy tissue, then the tissue becomes weakened, not only losing its structural integrity but opening the way for oxidative stress to do its mischief. People with a risk of cardiovascular disease will benefit from understanding the relationship between the damage done by homocysteine and the protection afforded by antioxidants.

3. The behavior of homocysteine actually liberates free radicals to do their mischief, reminding us that the external environment is not the exclusive source of oxidative damage. Consider what would happen if you, captivated by Queen Methionine, decided to eat lots of protein or take supplements of methionine so that you would have plenty of methyls to maintain your DNA. If you happen to be a person with weak mechanisms for transforming homocysteine to its job in the sanitation department or back into methionine you will unleash homocysteine on your chemistry and do yourself harm. About one third of individuals with cardiovascular disease have a tendency to the damage produced by high levels of homocysteine.[23] If you have a personal or family history of vascular disease, it would be a factor (among others)* to weigh in assessing your situation.

Use the following test to measure your homocysteine level: Eat meat, poultry, eggs, fish or beans at every meal for 24 hours or take a methionine supplement, 250 mg four times in 24 hours, while you collect a 24-hour urine specimen for measurement of homocysteine. Alternatively, you could have a blood specimen taken at the end of the 24-hour period for homocysteine measurement. An abnormally high level calls for a trial of folic acid and, perhaps, vitamin $B_6$ and $B_{12}$ supplementation followed by repeated testing to confirm your success in removing homocysteine from your body. Once the test is done, you will need to understand that a high intake of protein, with its load of homocysteine, may be beneficial or harmful depending on how well you have taken care of your homocysteine problem with the vitamin supplements that suit your particular quirk.

Stamler and Slivka speculate that pacifying homocysteine in individuals with high levels may be also accomplished with various

---

* Such as a need for extra magnesium, a need for more unsaturated fatty acids, and, of course, a tendency to high cholesterol levels.

substances, including feverfew extract, that permit covering the sticky sulfur with a nitrogen-bearing group.

4. Next, if you are wondering why such a toxic transformation of methionine should exist at all, the answer is that homocysteine is needed to make methionine's most useful metabolite, reduced glutathione (RG). RG is the most important worker in the detoxification department, the resupplier of vitamin E. In fact, detoxification is the most important activity in the body's biochemistry. Getting rid of toxins that come in from the outside, whether it be lead, mercury, arsenic or a variety of toxic chemicals; dumping used chemicals that are generated in our own chemistry; and detoxifying nasty substances that come from the germs that inhabit our intestines is the body's biggest consumer of energy for making new molecules. Reduced glutathione is a peptide made of three amino acids of which one, cysteine, is produced from homocysteine. The other two are glycine and glutamic acid. Peptides are abundant in your cells. Many message-carrying molecules such as ACTH and endorphins are peptides. RG is the most abundant and widely distributed peptide of them all and it has many jobs, most of them having to do with protecting you from oxidative damage and detoxification. It also works on several construction crews, synthesizing or forming larger molecules out of smaller ones. The most important thing to remember about RG's activities is that when RG detoxifies substances that are produced by your own metabolism (domestic waste, so to speak), it is able to transport the unwanted molecules to the outside and then return for another load. If, however, the toxic load is from the external environment (lead, cadmium or mercury for example), then RG has to take the load to the dump and stay there, never to return. RG is expensive; its presence depends on a metabolically costly and potentially dangerous means of production. The result is that for every atom of toxic substances that you consume and later need to get rid of, you are asking reduced glutathione to take a one-way trip to the dump.

5. Finally RG has another job: tending a fire that is needed to create important messenger molecules called leukotrienes. Its job at the dump and protecting molecules from free radicals gives it an in-

sider's understanding of the dangers of oxidation. RG directs one of the few operations in which oxidative forces are needed to create a new molecule.

Meanwhile, back at the Royal Court, we were in the process of seeing how Queen Methionine could regain her sovereignty by getting the methyl she gave up through her activities in the guise of SAM. Remember that SAM is busy distributing methyls around the body and, in particular, with the help of folic acid, to DNA where the methyls are needed for synthesis and repair. The restoration of methionine from homocysteine now depends on folic acid, working in conjunction with vitamin $B_{12}$ and vitamin $B_6$. A lack of sufficient amounts of folic acid to accomplish this task implies a dual threat to your organism. The first is the potential for the build-up of homocysteine and the second is the potential for insufficient folic acid to repair DNA with the consequence of chromosome damage. Cancer arises in tissues that are busy being constantly renewed, such as the mucous membrane of the lungs and the digestive, urinary and reproductive tracts when the supply of reparative methyls fails for lack of the B vitamin, folic acid.[24]

It is probably not helpful, however, to keep focusing on cancer as the risk to be avoided. There are plenty of other things that can go wrong long before something turns into cancer. The implications for functional impairment in cognition, reproduction and vitality in general are likely to be more widespread than the risk of cancer per se. Current medical technology does not have very good ways of measuring the impairment. The reason for covering this fairly complex branch of the chemistry of detoxification and repair is that it will become the hot new issue over the next few years. It has a bearing on the two major chronic illnesses of our culture: cardiovascular disease and malignancies. It is more important than cholesterol; however detoxification is at the same stage as was cholesterol research 20 years ago. Eventually, the cholesterol research led to the development of drugs to lower cholesterol, and the medical profession was educated by the pharmaceutical industry to take a sharper look at cholesterol as a risk factor for cardiovascular disease. Problems of homocysteine and related chemistry will turn out to be more important to illness prevention than cholesterol ever was, but at the moment and for the foreseeable future the main remedies for individuals with the problem are nutritional supplements. This bodes poorly for patients in a medical environment that still categorizes nutrients as wimpy compared to pharmaceuticals.

# CHAPTER 10

# Peptides from Foods:

## Molecular Masquerade

Wʜᴇɴ ᴍᴏsᴛ ғᴏʟᴋs ʜᴇᴀʀ the term detoxification they think of individuals who are addicted to alcohol, cocaine, opium and its derivatives, barbiturates, benzodiazepines (such as Valium®) or other hard drugs. Detoxification for such people involves the same kind of chemistry we have been discussing with regard to getting rid of unwanted substances from the body. There is, however, an added feature that makes the process more difficult. The addict's chemistry has gotten used to the addictive substance, the presence of which allows him or her to feel relatively normal even though it may be doing significant mischief over all. The absence of the substance creates a toxic state that is quite different from what we have been discussing. It has to do with receptor sites. The lock on your front door is a receptor site. More appropriately, the key to turn off an alarm system is one, too. The alarm is set to go off under certain circumstances unless you put in the key and turn it. An impending state of excitement has been quenched by the necessary presence of the key. The receptor site is "happy," so to speak. In living systems there is a mechanism of adaptation in which cells change in response to how much of a particular stimulus they receive. The more opium is presented over a period of time, the more receptor sites are created to accept the opium. In the case of opium, the adaptation is particularly poignant because the narcotic molecules in the opium work because they closely resemble peptides we use in our own nervous and immune systems. In fact, opium was known long before anyone was aware of the endorphins we produce in our own chemistry for the modulation of a myriad of nervous and immune functions. When endorphins were discovered, they were named for the morphine-like molecules from opium that resemble them. The whole set of them are called opioids, and they are all peptides.

If it were a question of just saying no to drugs, the matter would be simple. Mark Martini's story illustrates how complicated things can get. His birth was normal at 37 weeks gestation. He was put under lights to bleach out the yellow color of his jaundice (another form of detoxification). Could this be an early warning that he was not as well-equipped in the detoxification department as other babies? Mark was breast-fed briefly, then switched to formula. His first DPT shot gave rise to local inflammation with a swollen leg, and he screamed for hours. At four months of age, after his second immunization, which was changed to leave out the pertussis, he developed a cough and congestion and was given an antibiotic. After that he was on antibiotics three times in his first year; from his second to fourth year he was on antibiotics 17 times. He had surgery at age two for hernia and was hospitalized for a rotovirus infection shortly thereafter. On each of these two occasions he had intravenous antibiotics. He stopped speech development after the hernia. When his delayed development was evaluated he underwent a number of studies to rule out a seizure disorder and was then diagnosed as autistic.

When Mark was given a treatment to reverse the changes in his bowel germs that were wrought by the antibiotics he developed a better attention span, but he remained in a state of altered perception of the world around him; he had an increased sensitivity to all kinds of stimulation and was preoccupied by the self-stimulation of various repetitive gestures, movements and noises. He became especially sensitive to tastes and smells. He was extremely fussy about foods and would have gladly subsisted on French fries and ginger ale if they were provided. He seemed intrigued by some odors and unusually aversive to others, such as certain perfumes. He covered his ears when confronted by the whine of a vacuum cleaner or the hum of the air conditioner.

Mark's blood test for food allergies showed reactions to 26 foods out of the more than 90 tested. I decided that it would be better to discover the basis for his immune system's attitude toward food and try to repair that than to embark on the unfeasible and unhealthy further restriction of his diet. After trying various approaches to his problem he was faring better but was still a boy with global developmental handicaps. I had glimpses that there was a smart boy inside of Mark who could emerge if the perceptual chaos of his senses and immune system could get straightened out. His family carried out a strenuous program of reaching out to him and insisting that he take the very difficult steps involved in pulling together his own resources.

In the meantime I met Karl Reichelt, M.D., Ph.D., the director of Clinical Chemistry in the Department of Pediatric Research at The National Hospital in Oslo, Norway. Our meeting occurred at a brainstorming conference aimed at accelerating the course of research in autism and related problems. The meeting was held under the auspices of The Autism Research Institute under the leadership of Bernard Rimland, Ph.D. who, in 1965, wrote the book[25] that immediately altered the landscape in which autism had previously been viewed as an emotional disorder resulting from poor parenting on the part of "refrigerator mothers." Dr. Rimland, himself the parent of an autistic child, denounced the prevailing dogma, challenging it with sufficient data to convince reasonable people to abandon the old dogma. It would be found, Dr. Rimland wrote, that autism is a biologic disorder with aspects that resemble a state of intoxication, confusion of the senses and abnormal processing of stimuli. Dr. Rimland soon became the center of a huge network of parents and began collecting information from them as to what worked or did not work to help their children. The collective impatience with the pace of research gave rise to the conference where I met Dr. Reichelt as well as another prominent peptide researcher, Paul Shattock, Ph.D., Senior Lecturer in Pharmacy at the School of Health Sciences at University of Sunderland, in England. Dr. Reichelt and Dr. Shattock have each made observations following work begun by Dr. F. C. Dohan[26-29] in the 1960s based on the observed patterns of certain kinds of severe disturbances of perception and thinking that correlated with the consumption of cereal grains. I had taken many patients off of gluten-containing grains (wheat, rye, barley and probably oats), but not until meeting Dr. Reichelt did I move such a consideration up on my list of things to try for autistic children. Then I took it from the back burner and made it a prime therapeutic priority.

I sent Mark's urine to Norway for Dr. Reichelt to analyze. The result showed that the urine contained abnormal peptides that came from certain foods and had passed undigested into Mark's blood. This damaging substance was not a venom, a poorly detoxified hormone, a product of fermentative activities of the bowel flora, an allergen or a substance that has been damaged by oxidative changes. These mischievous molecules were digested from the normal protein of normal food up to a point, but unfortunately for Mark, they escaped the last few steps in a digestive process that ordinarily reduces the thousands of amino acids joined in a protein into separate individual amino acids.

Recall that an amino acid is a small molecule that may function independently as the raw material for making thyroid hormone, various neurotransmitters and other important message carriers in biochemistry. All but one (taurine) of the 22 amino acids found in nature can be combined in small numbers to form peptides or in large numbers to form proteins. The digestive process breaks down protein molecules into shorter and shorter segments, the ultimate goal being the liberation of single amino acids that are absorbed as such into the bloodstream where they are used as raw materials. If the digestive process is incomplete and/or there is a leakiness of the intestinal wall separating the intestinal contents from the bloodstream, short segments of several amino acids (peptides) may enter the blood. These peptides join other peptides in the blood and tissues that the body has made to carry messages from place to place in the body.

Considering that many different peptides may enter the bloodstream as a result of incomplete digestion of various foods, there exists the possibility that the outside (exogenous) peptides may be mistaken in the body's communication systems for inside (endogenous) peptides. Exogenous peptides that may cause mischief by being mistaken for endorphins and other endogenous peptides are called exorphins. Observations made years ago by Dr. F. C. Dohan have led to more recent evidence[30-40] that peptides from gluten (one of the principal proteins in wheat and other grains) and casein (one of the main proteins in the milk of all mammals) may be particularly mischievous in producing unwanted endorphin-like effects in certain susceptible individuals. Dr. Reichelt's thorough bibliography on the relationship between peptides, digestive function and permeability, food antigens, neurochemistry and the dietary and neuroleptic treatment of autistic persons and others is included in the references.[41]

After obtaining results showing abnormal peptides from gluten in grains and casein from any cow's milk product, I proposed that Mark be taken off all sources of gluten and dairy, and his family did so. He refused to eat any food at all, he barely slept and he was in a constant state of nervous hyperactivity, bounding from place to place only to interrupt his turmoil with episodes of biting and hitting. He refused to drink and would have become dehydrated if liquids had not been forced on him. The good news was that for the first time in his life he consistently formed bowel movements and became more interested in exercising bowel control.

After the first few days of this, I had two questions. 1) What was going on? and 2) How could I prevent Mark from becoming undernourished? As an answer to the second question, I recommended a supplement of a rice-protein-based, nutrient-dense food supplement plus flaxseed oil as sources of calories and good fats that could be added to his juice and which he could be coaxed to swallow. What seemed to be going on was withdrawal, a common feature of abstinence from addictive foods or substances. We expect withdrawal symptoms when coffee is given up because we know it contains the drug caffeine. We generally assume that ordinary foods do not contain "drugs," but a basic point of this chapter is to question that assumption. Mark's suffering continued for several weeks, during which time I was able to see him while attending a conference in the Midwest near his home. At this point I had predicted the imminent end of his ordeal many times. I knew that when I saw him I should consider any measures that might finally lessen his problems. When I met with Mark and his family, we agreed that there were only two explanations for what was going on. One was that he was angry with us for taking him off two foods that had been an important part of his diet and that his plight represented a kind of hunger strike. The other was that the receptor sites in his nervous system were still crying out to be soothed with the endorphin-like peptides from milk and gluten. The same peptides presumably had caused confusion in his chemistry, inducing the altering of his perceptions, mood, thinking and behavior, but such negative effects would not necessarily preclude a tranquilizing effect that was missed when the peptides were withdrawn.

Had any other kind of treatment produced the reaction we saw in Mark, his family and I would have stopped it long before the five weeks that had passed before I saw him in my hotel room. But withdrawing something is different from adding something. I could not conceive of reintroducing gluten and casein into his diet because of the knowledge gained from Dr. Reichelt's tests (in addition to knowing from previous tests that Mark had high levels of antibodies to milk and wheat, as well as the specific proteins, casein and gluten). Mark had lost about 15 pounds. He was in constant motion and lost in his autism. I made a few suggestions that I thought might help hasten the end of an ordeal that I had given up predicting: more activated charcoal and more alkaline salts, the only two cure-alls that I have discovered in 30 years of doctoring.

Activated charcoal is a medicinal form of charcoal that has the capacity to absorb whatever molecules it encounters. The simple measure of supplying charcoal to the digestive tract not only accomplishes its advertised digestive intent of absorbing gas and toxins there, but it appears to aid detoxification anywhere in the body. Presumably the reduction of toxins accomplished by the short-term use of activated charcoal takes some pressure off the whole detoxification system by diminishing the burden from the gut. Activated charcoal is indiscriminate in what it absorbs. Therefore it should not be taken with food or medicines as it would absorb them, too, and it should not be taken for long periods of time. It is, however, good for whatever ails you, as are alkaline salts, sold as Alka-Seltzer *without* aspirin. This form of Alka-Seltzer, which comes in a gold package and is nicknamed Alka Gold by doctors who know the value of alkaline salts, contains only sodium and potassium bicarbonate; it is one step up from the baking soda found in any kitchen, which is just sodium bicarbonate and will do in a pinch.

Basically healthy people can take an Alka Gold or a half-teaspoon of baking soda in a glass of water when they are feeling very hungry and irritable to the point of becoming quite bad company, or have premenstrual syndrome, or a hangover or are coming down with a cold and they will almost certainly feel better. It is best not to do so on a very full stomach or if the kidneys or lungs don't work well. In nearly every instance in which people feel sick, they tend to get slightly acidic. Every day the body needs to get rid of smoke and ashes from the metabolic fire and nearly always there is extra acid that constitutes the most fundamental problem in detoxification. When just about anything goes wrong with the body there is a transient tendency to become acidic, and by sending some alkali through the system, the body has a chance to recover balance.

Mark got substantial temporary relief by taking repeated doses of the Alka Gold and finally, after six weeks of misery, he turned the corner. I don't know if it was because of the charcoal and the Alka Gold, because I gave him an old-fashioned antihistamine that tends to stimulate appetite (cyprohepatadine) or because his withdrawal finally ran its course. Mark emerged from the ordeal a changed boy. Like many autistic children he made major leaps in his behavior and cognitive abilities.

The withdrawal symptoms that Mark experienced are unusual but illustrate the opioid addiction and withdrawal connection to the problem. Most autistic children, as well as others who may benefit from avoiding these foods, experience improvement within days, although the improvement may continue for months after embarking on such a treatment because the peptides are washed out of the body slowly and the nervous system takes time to heal.

Mark's withdrawal was more difficult and he got less benefit than other children I know who have gone from being wild and disoriented to almost completely normal within weeks of eliminating gluten and casein from their diets. Observing diverse and impressive changes in patients avoiding gluten and casein leads me to the following thought. All food contains at least some protein and all proteins yield at least some peptides even when they are properly digested. Every person absorbs not only the small molecules liberated at the end of perfect digestion but a substantial quantity of larger ones including not only peptides but proteins as well. Many people have intestines that are leaky, permitting excess absorption of unwanted molecules. It seems to me that what we observe in peptide-sensitive autistic children has implications that will turn up in other ways in the future. Over the next decade more and more troublesome peptides will be found to cause problems in all of the many areas of human chemistry where normal peptides carry out the body's business, particularly in the brain and immune system.

# CHAPTER 11

# Dirty Smoke:

## Genetic Mistakes and Metabolic Abnormalities

In June of 1996 William Shaw, Ph.D., head of the toxicology lab of a major mid-western children's medical center was fired from his job because he presented his research findings at an international meeting attended by more than 100 physicians interested in the immunology and toxicology of autism and related disorders. The research he presented had already been presented previously at various scientific and medical meetings, and his findings had been published in a peer review scientific journal. I believe that his discoveries will lead to major breakthroughs in our understanding of many illnesses that go far beyond the field of children's developmental problems where Dr. Shaw made his first observations. It is hard to beat the injustice done to Dr. McCully when he pursued research in homocysteine to say nothing of several other recent medical "heretics" such as Dr. Barry Marshall, the discoverer of the germ, *Helicobacter pylori,* which causes stomach ulcers and other digestive problems, but Dr. Shaw's treatment was even worse. At our conference in Chicago he could not even present all of his data because his research files and some of his teaching slides were confiscated. Today Dr. Shaw is pursuing his research at Great Plains Laboratory in Overland Park, Kansas.

Here is the background on Dr. Shaw's research. A metabolic fire burns in each of us and the smoke from that fire is acid. A match burns a little dirtier than a candle, and our metabolic fire burns even dirtier because it takes place at a lower temperature. This is the main reason that we have to spend a lot of energy getting rid of the waste materials from our metabolism: they cannot be rendered into clean smoke and ashes. The breath we exhale constitutes the elimination of a certain burden of acid. What occurs in that process is the undoing of the reverse process that occurs in plants as they are exposed to the sun. Capturing sunlight, they make molecules of sugar (then starch) or fat by using the sun's energy to join carbon atoms from carbon dioxide in the air. Putting the carbon atoms together takes energy, and when we disassemble the sugars and fats of plants in our metabolism, we get the sun's energy back again for our metabolic use. Carbon dioxide is returned to the air as we make helpfully destructive use of free radicals supplied as oxygen in the air we breathe to rip the electrons off of our food molecules. The carbon dioxide we exhale is part of the smoke produced from our metabolic fire, and the ashes consist of various nonvolatile elements in our food, such as minerals. Because the fire burns at a very low temperature as compared with a candle flame, some of the smoke cannot be rendered (oxidized) to the point of being volatile and still exists in a form that can only be dissolved in the blood and thus transferred to the bile or urine to be discharged from the body. The substances that make up this nonvolatile "smoke" are still acid in nature. They derive from living or organic processes and they are called organic acids. To the extent that they represent the products of a fire that is not burning clean, they are "dirty smoke."

You can experience the effects of dirty smoke in your body by trying to run farther than you are really able to. At a certain point, your inadequately trained muscles will cramp up as they accumulate organic acids resulting from a poor balance between the supply of fuel and oxygen. In effect, it is the result of a fire that is burning at poor efficiency. Some of us are born with errors in the chemistry that constitutes the "disassembly line" of the metabolic fire in which sugar (glucose) and other molecules are taken apart to retrieve the sun's energy that is stored there.

## THE GENETIC ERROR IN SAMANTHA'S METABOLISM

When I was Chief Resident in Pediatrics at Yale, a child named Samantha was admitted on a few occasions with vomiting and lethargy and acidosis. In the first stages of such an illness there would be no reason to think of it as anything more than a "virus" that could be managed by watchful waiting and careful attention to the child's need to avoid dehydration during a temporary period of low intake. This child, however, became very sick, and her sister had died of a similar illness. Understandably, she was treated with caution and, as it happened, evaluated with the brilliance of Dr. Leon Rosenberg, who would later go on to become an international figure in the field of genetically-transmitted metabolic diseases and then Dean of Yale Medical School. Unlike many of us who kept biochemistry carefully balanced in our brains only until we passed the exams, Dr. Rosenberg had a clear picture of all the assembly and disassembly lines that comprise our chemistry. Ten years later I realized that I could not practice medicine without recapturing my own clear picture, but at the time I was up to my neck in the day-to-day operations of the pediatric service and was not directly involved in the care of Samantha or the untangling of her mysterious problems. Little did I understand at the time that the biochemistry of rare and "exotic" conditions is often the tip of the iceberg in common conditions that I would encounter for the rest of my life as a physician. As you will see, Samantha's problem touches on a branch of biochemistry that in her represented a singular case, but which also pointed to a crossroad in biochemistry that is basic to understanding the care and feeding of our bodies.

A particular organic acid turned up to account for her acidic condition. Its presence was due to a wrong step in the disassembly line in which a particular amino acid (valine) is prepared for being discarded and burned up in her body's furnace, the so-called citric acid or Krebs cycle. As the amino acid is dismantled its name changes with the loss of various parts so that at a certain point it becomes known as methylmalonic acid. Its next transformation, in which it is diminished further, was faulty in Samantha, and as a consequence the methylmalonic acid became stuck, so to speak, and constituted a build-up of dirty smoke that poisoned her and produced an illness with excessive vomiting and lethargy such as children get from many different causes.

There are only so many ways of *being* sick, but there are many ways of *getting* sick. The misstep in Samantha's chemistry is one in which several molecules participate as helpers in the disassembly step. Among these helpers is one big molecule, an enzyme, that Samantha simply could not make properly because the gene in her chromosomes did not carry the right instructions for her to produce it correctly. She was born that way. Another of the helpers in the step is vitamin $B_{12}$. It has two jobs in all of human biochemistry and one of them is to help the enzyme drag a methyl group off of the methylmalonic acid so that it becomes ready to take its place in the furnace with its new name, succinic acid, which is a part of a disassembled glucose molecule as it is getting burned for its energy. Dr. Rosenberg found that Samantha's problem could be substantially repaired by having her take very large amounts of vitamin $B_{12}$. Even though her enzyme did not work at all well, supplying very large amounts of $B_{12}$ took care of the problem to the extent of saving Samantha's life without having actually produced a cure. Rosenberg coauthored a major text[42] describing Samantha's metabolic errors and scores of others, some of which may be corrected in a similar fashion with the addition of large amounts of vitamins. At the end of his book he speculated thoughtfully about the pace at which metabolic disorders were discovered and the potential for misunderstanding and misusing vitamins based on their importance in treating a few individuals with rare conditions.

"We have proof," cautioned Rosenberg and coauthor, Dr. C. R. Scriver, "that for *some* persons in *particular* circumstances, pharmacologic doses of vitamins are essential. But should we generalize from the specific data in a few special circumstances? We believe that such generalizations *are* being made but without the benefit of evidence equivalent to that obtained in the vitamin-responsive inborn errors of metabolism" (their emphasis). This opinion springs from a viewpoint that sees people as normal unless they have a disease. The prevailing attitude of modern medicine is the same now as when I was trained in the 1960s: People become sick because they get a disease. The attitude cultivates a sense that we are all potential victims of some kind of attack that just sort of happens. More and more, we are finding that our genetic makeup is quite decisive as to what kind of disease we get so that blame gets put onto our ancestors. Thus we are made to feel more and more helpless to avoid a fate that is cast in our genes.

An alternative way of thinking is to accept that each of us has a distinctive immunologic and biochemical makeup. Consequently, all of us have inborn errors of metabolism (usually very mild as compared to Samantha) and thus nearly all of us must learn to tailor our diet, nutritional supplements, physical and social environment to match our individual needs and to make the best of our genetic endowment. This alternative to current mainstream medicine focuses on balance within the individual as contrasted to treatment of a disease. I will return to the subject in chapter 17.

Back to Samantha. Samantha was poisoned by smoke from her own fire. Her problem was diagnosed by detecting a normal organic acid that appeared in her urine in excessive amounts because of an inherited problem with the disassembly line that we all use to burn any extra amount of a particular amino acid that is a normal (and substantial) part of everyone's diet. Dr. Rosenberg showed brilliance in identifying Samantha's problem, although his method (analysis of a patient's urine for the presence of abnormal organic acids) was already a standard tool in medicine at the time. Samantha's treatment involved limiting the amount of valine in her diet (which is difficult because valine is one of the most abundant amino acids in all proteins) and megadoses of vitamin $B_{12}$. In the current medical paradigm Samantha was a victim of a rare disease, and most of the rest of us can feel lucky that we don't have such a disease. In an alternative paradigm, we are all metabolically different and, while most of us get along just fine, we have access to the same kinds of tools that were used to diagnose Samantha's disease to find our own more subtle sorts of imbalances. If we are well and wish to look for ways to remain so, or if we are sick—with or without a diagnosis—these tools can help us address those imbalances, quite possibly making a substantial difference in our future well-being. The attitude we bring to the use of these tools can make a crucial difference in the outcome of their results. If our attitude is disease-oriented, we may come up empty. If, on the other hand, our attitude centers on the concept of balance—finding something that we need more or less of to help our biochemistry and immune/nervous systems work more efficiently—we are likely to find an effective treatment for the prevention of future illness by taking supplements of substances that are a natural part of the body's makeup or by avoiding or ridding ourselves of toxins and allergens.

## OTHER GENETIC MISTAKES

Now we have the background with which to return to Dr. Shaw. Some years ago he worked as a biochemist in a laboratory where his research involved identifying the germ causing an infection in a given patient by examining the person's blood, urine or other body fluid for the "smoke" from the germ's fire. Some years later Dr. Shaw was the head of a laboratory performing the same kinds of analyses used to detect Samantha's problem as well as hundreds of other kinds of metabolic abnormalities whose signature is abnormal organic acids in the blood or urine. Dr. Shaw noted that the urine of some children with developmental problems had excessive amounts of organic acids that did not come from the child but were by-products of the metabolism of the germs inhabiting the intestine of the child. Such organic acids had been noticed by others in the past, and the prevailing opinion in medicine was basically: "Those are microbial metabolites (e.g., germ chemicals) and they are not what we are looking for (e.g., people chemicals); thus, they are not important.

The point is that there are really two fires in each of us. One is our own fire, or our metabolism, which may or may not burn dirty. The other produces a collective "smoke" of metabolic by-products from all the infinitesimal fires of the germs inhabiting our digestive tract. Much of this smoke passes from our gut with the bowel movements and gas that we pass. Some of it, however, is absorbed into our body and must then be detoxified and excreted just as if we had consumed it in some other way. Perhaps there is something in this smoke that disagrees with us; perhaps we might be especially sensitive to these organic acids and the other toxins that keep them company.

What kinds of toxins might these be? Might they be strange toxins such as those that come from a venomous tick? Might they be like alcohol? Might they be hormone-like? Might they be allergens, so that one person but not another could get hives from one or more of them? Because they are organic acids, might they look so much like our own organic acid that they would wend their way into our metabolism and screw things up along the same lines as the peptides can? Yes. Yes. Yes. Yes. Yes.

Dr. Shaw's work is very recent,[43,44] and as I write this he has just opened a new lab to continue the work for which he was censured by his hospital's hierachy. The reason for telling you about his work is to ask you to think about the implications and watch as his ideas develop over the next few years. As you will see in the next chapter, there is other evidence to support these ideas and, if you understand their implications, there are things you can do now that will reduce your risk of ill health while continuing to watch from the sidelines. Here is how the microbial organic acid picture looks now and how it will develop.


## THE IMPACT OF ANTIBIOTICS ON METABOLISM

Jeffrey Smith was admitted repeatedly to the hospital where Dr. Shaw worked, with seizures caused by very low blood sugar levels. The seizures started after Jeffrey was given antibiotics for a strep throat at nine months of age. He had been completely well until that time. His problem remained a mystery over several months, and several admissions to the hospital where all kinds of tests were done did not reveal a clue within the usual framework of understanding the regulation of blood sugar. His insulin levels were never more than 20 percent above normal, not enough to explain his danger-ously low levels of blood glucose. In the course of time Jeffrey's doctors ordered several tests of his organic acid profile for the nor-mal reasons, i.e., to see Jeffrey's metabolic by-products. The lab results revealed very large amounts of a compound that clearly did not come from Jeffrey, but from the germs in his bowel. The com-pound was not, technically speaking, an organic acid but a kind of sugar that is made by germs in the fungus (mold, mildew, yeast) realm that were somewhere in Jeffrey's body. Dr. Shaw knew that this compound could be made to disappear from Jeffrey's urine by giving him nystatin, a medicine that kills yeasts in the intestine but does not enter the bloodstream and so is without risk. He mentioned this to Jeffrey's doctors each time Jeffrey was readmitted to the hos-pital and was retested in his lab, but to no avail. The communication from Jeffrey's doctors went something like this: "We want you to look for all possible metabolic diseases, but don't keep telling us about that yeast nonsense." As Dr. Shaw tells the story, he finally became more aggressive with his observations. After all, he pointed out, the levels of the compound in Jeffrey's urine were extremely high and since it was a kind of sugar, it certainly might disturb Jeffrey's sugar metabolism. This persistence led to Shaw's being put on probation at the hospital. He was instructed not to report infor-mation about microbial organic acids unless specifically requested to do so. Eventually, Jeffrey was given a treatment with nystatin, the medicine to kill the yeasts. The abnormal sugar in his urine dropped from measurements in the thousands to close to zero, his blood sugar rose to normal and his seizures stopped. Jeffrey's health prob-lems had all begun after a course of antibiotics.

Jeffrey's case is unusual in its severity, but I think it exemplifies a phenomenon that is widespread and that has to do with the effects of altering bowel flora with antibiotics. Dr. Shaw's research focuses on abnormal organic acids found in children with developmental problems. My take on it is that such children are, to the medical profession, like the canaries miners used to take into the mine as an early warning for toxic air. Some children with developmental prob-lems are very sensitive. I have tried to understand their biochemistry and immunology for the sake of sorting out their problems. While doing so I have learned things that apply to all of us in ways that affect how we think about underlying mechanisms for all sorts of illnesses, especially those in which the immune and central nervous systems are involved. In particular it makes me realize how essential it is to protect the core of essential cells in our immune and central nervous systems by protecting the communication systems of our chemistry. The most subtle danger to our chemistry comes from molecules that, like the peptides discussed previously, so resemble our own molecules that they blend in with the crowd and go unnoticed until it turns out that they not only cannot function as do the molecules they mimic, but they occupy strategic spaces in our chemistry and interfere with our own molecules. This is a key point for all of us who have a natural inclination to fear things that appear strange or outlandish. If we conjure up a picture of toxins as mostly weird and alien chemicals we may fail to understand that mimicry is one of nature's most pervasive tricks. The viceroy butterfly who mimics the toxic monarch in order to borrow from the latter's poisonous reputation among predator birds is a good example of the creative uses of mimicry. A random molecule that interferes with the way your molecule works because it looks just like it reminds us that in this sense we have more to fear from friendly looking chemicals than from monstrous ones.


## DANGEROUS MASQUERADERS

Most of the children Dr. Shaw has studied do not have serious blood sugar problems. They have problems with perception, language and attention that place their diagnosis in the autism spectrum of disorders. In most instances their urine organic acid analysis shows the same sugar that bothered Jeffrey—in lower but still abnormal concentrations—and a few compounds that closely resemble one of two categories of human molecules: neurotransmitters and citric-acid-cycle intermediaries. Recall that the citric acid cycle is the biochemical machinery in which glucose molecules are disassembled to release energy. The disassembly proceeds stepwise, and at each stage a new and smaller molecule is formed. It is a cycle because the fragment that is left at the end of the process is stuck back onto the one that begins the process and then goes around again. As the cycle proceeds certain molecules are formed in the fire that have multiple uses elsewhere in the body, so they are retrieved, snatched from the fire, so to speak, for other uses. Interference with the metabolic fire can, then, not only result in an inefficient energy production, but the raw materials needed for other body processes may run short. What other body process is heavily dependent on raw materials for making new molecules? Detoxification! The sanitation department is the energy department's biggest consumer.

One of the compounds that Dr. Shaw kept turning up is called 3-oxoglutaric acid. It is a very close look-alike to 2-oxoglutaric acid (also called alpha-ketoglutarate or AKG). The two molecules resemble each other so closely that one could be easily mistaken for the other, especially since the 3-oxoglutaric is a fungus chemical and the body really has no experience with it. Dr. Shaw says it is analogous to coming home without the key to unlock the front door. You find a key that looks like your key and it fits into the lock. You give it a good try and it breaks off in the lock. Now you have a worse problem than when you started. The analogy adequately describes the effect of having interference from look-alike molecules. It cannot adequately explain the possible consequences of having a molecule masquerade as AKG. Interfering with its role in the citric acid cycle is bad enough. In addition, of all the multi-use molecules in the body, AKG is the champ. AKG is everywhere helping to rearrange, build and take molecules apart. If you were to look down on your biochemical municipality from overhead you would get the idea that AKG, SAM (S-adenosyl methionine) and reduced glutathione are like the taxi cabs, buses and subways of New York City. Now imagine slipping into the city a fleet of yellow cars that look like taxis and let you get in but never let you get out. That would be a problem.

Look-alike molecules are not new to the thinking of doctors. Most drugs work on that principle. Many antibiotics work by fooling the germ into thinking the drug is useful because it resembles one of the germ's own. Many cancer drugs work by getting cancer cells (as well, unfortunately, as normal ones) to build a close look-alike into their DNA molecules, which then cannot function normally and result in the cells' death.

The idea that intestinal germs produce toxins that result in illness is also an old one. A century ago the discovery of the multitude of germs in the human gut led to the notion (proposed by Metchnikoff, Pasteur's successor as director of the Pasteur Institute) that these germs must be the root of most illness. The idea got out of hand so that enemas became, in the popular mind and practice, an overused method to cleanse the bowel of potential trouble engendered by all the "bad germs." By the time I went to medical school this notion had been vigorously discredited by a medical profession alarmed at the potential for enemas and other forms of preoccupation with "regularity" to cause trouble, not the least of which was psychological, in children who became victims of their parents' fixation. It is harder for a discredited idea to be revived than for a new idea to gain acceptance. The accumulating evidence that intestinal germs have a complex interaction with our chemistry will regain medical recognition soon. Moreover, the effects of intestinal germs provoke reactions in individuals that may vary considerably from person to person, sometimes masquerading as known autoimmune, allergic and chronic inflammatory diseases affecting a particular body system or organ.

Dr. Shaw's work has shown us that some individuals, particularly children with autism, have very large amounts of di-hydroxyphenylpropionic acid in their urine and that this molecule is made by certain bacteria, not fungi, in the intestine. Most of the children I have treated to remove the di-hydroxyphenylpropionic acid by killing the germs have not improved the same way they would by killing the fungi that produce other organic acids, even when the levels of the di-hydroxyphenylpropionic acid fall by a hundred-fold. Thus far then, this look-alike to a neurotransmitter is just an example of the way that intestinal germs can produce molecules that resemble our own. Going by present knowledge, we have good reason to try to keep a healthy normal population of germs thriving in our intestine. They say that a pregnant woman is eating for two, herself and her fetus. You may not be pregnant, but you are eating for 10,000,000,000,000: you and all the germs that inhabit your gut.

CHAPTER 12

# Dietary Fiber and Hormone Regulation

WHAT DO THE GERMS of your intestine like to eat? They will eat just about anything, but dietary fiber feeds good intestinal germs which discourage unfavorable ones. I can think of few other topics in medicine that have flip-flopped as has fiber. In my training I was taught that fiber was a useless, inert ingredient in our foods and we should all look forward to the day when, like the astronauts, we could subsist on some sort of highly refined goop that provided us with just the right ingredients for physiologic prosperity. Out of Africa came Dr. Dennis Burkitt, who, while practicing medicine in Uganda, noticed that Africans eating a traditional diet had a completely different pattern of illness than those people, including those of African descent, eating a Western diet. The dietary content of roughage, fiber or indigestible cellulose that makes up the main structural component of plants is what accounted for the fact that Africans were spared most of the diseases that affect us, from diabetes and heart disease to appendicitis and hemorrhoids. My own African experience gave me first hand exposure to Dr. Burkitt's ideas.

Of the many ways that fiber promotes good health, such as providing bulk and holding water plus the many positive influences

on dozens of problems from acne to ulcers,[45] there is one you probably have not heard about. This one should open your mind to the
cybernetic factors linking diet, the germs that live in your intestine,
antibiotics, hormone balance and cancers of the reproductive organs
such as breast and prostate. From time to time we hear that a particular substance has been declared safe or unsafe based on whether or
not it causes cancer or at least leads to mutations in the DNA of
living things, a marker for a cancer-causing potential. As you can
appreciate from the examples I have given, there are many ways that
an unwanted substance can bother a person that have nothing to do
with cancer, and in some ways the preoccupation with cancer tends
to put people off track. Even when preoccupied with cancer causa-
tion, I think we hear too much about environmental toxins as compared to ways we can enhance our repair mechanisms, such as those
involving folic acid, that enable us to keep our DNA fresh and un-
damaged. As you read on, I hope you will keep in mind that cancer
may be a more easily grasped and feared consequence of the chain of
events being described than, say, "hormone imbalance." When visiting a doctor a patient is much more likely to hear that the hormones
are a little out of balance than that he or she has cancer, yet this is
usually by way of saying that there is not any real problem and that
the imbalance "just happens" and is not really subject to remedy.
After all, it is not a "disease."

Imbalance, however, is the precursor of disease. Imbalance may
be associated with symptoms that a person or his or her physician
may deem "insignificant" because they do not constitute a disease.
However, imbalance worsens all illness as it progresses, even
when—in the case of trauma or infection—the illness may begin in a
person who is in a state of balance. A person with "insignificant"
symptoms of hormonal imbalance may take a special interest in the
evidence linking long term subtle effects of certain kinds of dietary
fiber with the ultimate effect of prostate and breast cancers.

For many years epidemiologists have recognized that the incidence of reproductive cancers (breast in women and prostate in
men) is much higher in populations consuming a Western diet as
compared to the vegetable-based diet consumed in most of Asia,

Africa and South America. The incidence of bowel cancer, cardiovascular disease and other problems varies in the same way.

Dr. Herman Adlercreutz (presently Professor of Clinical Chemistry at the University of Helsinki) developed a theory that something in fiber mediates the healthy effects of a vegetable-based diet. He was particularly intrigued by statistics that showed a low cancer incidence in Finns and others consuming a traditional rye bread that is made from the whole grain and leavened not with yeast but with a culture of *lactobacillus* (acidophilus)—the same kind of germ that ferments yogurt and sauerkraut. It appeared that consumption of rye bread was associated with an exceptionally low reproductive cancer incidence for Finns as compared with other Europeans who consume wheat bread. Dr. Adlercreutz's theories were not accepted by the scientific community when he first proposed them, as fiber was thought to be unnecessary or at least inert. It is understood that reproductive cancers are stimulated, after their inception, by higher levels of hormones (estrogen in women and testosterone in men) so that if, apart from any hormonal influence, such cancers appear, then factors that contribute to high hormone levels would favor the persistence and growth of such cancers. For his theories to be true there would have to be a substance present in, say rye fiber, that would do one of the following:

1. Inhibit high levels of sex hormones during the life of the individual so that in the event of a cancer arising, it would not be stimulated.
2. Limit the actual growth of cancer cells themselves.
3. Hinder the development of blood vessels that a cancer requires around itself for nourishment.

## CANCER-INHIBITING FOODS AND HOW THEY WORK

Dr. Adlercreutz and others have amassed convincing data showing that compounds called isoflavonoids and lignans isolated from rye fiber and soy protein and various other vegetable sources will modulate sex hormones, inhibit cancer growth and the nourishment of

cancers by surrounding blood vessels. The use of isolated compounds in research does not imply that the use of these compounds
as isolated substances will be forthcoming. There is a strong argument for the use of certain nutritional supplements as isolated compounds, e.g., folic acid. In the case of the fiber-derived compounds,
Dr. Adlercreutz points out that "it should be kept in mind that it is
to be preferred to consume original food, or food modified only
slightly, instead of consuming isolated or synthetic compounds."[46]

When someone eats a piece of whole rye bread, most of the
protein, carbohydrate and fat is digested in the stomach and small
intestine so that the available molecules of amino acids, sugars and
fats pass into the bloodstream, leaving behind a residue of material
that is carbohydrate in nature but resists digestive efforts to separate
the sugar molecules of which it is composed. It originally comes
from plant cells where it forms their walls. These walls are stiff and
sturdy as opposed to the flexible and delicate membranes of animal
cells. Cellulose is mashed but kept intact for the making of paper.
Cellulose molecules can be dissolved and manipulated to produce
celluloid and rayon, but they can only be digested into their component sugar molecules by bacteria. Such bacteria in the intestine of
my two goats are the only means they have of digesting their hay
and leaves, but we humans lack any such bacteria in our gut. We do
not have bacteria that liberate the component sugars from cellulose
so that we can burn the sugar for energy. The bacteria that we do
have, however, liberate substances from dietary fiber. We can then
absorb these compounds into our bodies. Certain bacteria of our
intestinal flora are the only way we have of extracting from fiber the
compounds that perform the three cancer-inhibiting functions noted
above. Dr. Adlerkreutz's research has shown the absence of such
compounds from the bowel and blood of individuals who have
taken antibiotics. The compounds stay absent for a prolonged time,
more than three months, so that if they were to take an antibiotic,
twice a year, they might inhibit the production of the cancer-
preventing compounds half of the time. The protective compounds
from soy do not need the mediating effects of bacteria, but can be
absorbed during digestion of the soy protein. Numerous experiments demonstrate correlations between levels of the substances

from rye fiber and soy protein (as well as from flaxseed, sesame seed, various grains and tea) and the growth and incidence of prostate and breast cancers in animals and in humans. The collective research in this area has been published in dozens of articles since the 1970s. Another decade may pass before specific recommendations emerge from the scientists who are most intimately involved in this research. Yet another decade may lapse before we hear official recommendations for dietary change or supplementation. In the meantime those of us who are familiar with the research may find it prudent to consume whole rye bread leavened with *lactobacillus* and to increase our intake of soy protein, tofu or miso soup. Obviously, those allergic to rye or soy must avoid these foods.

# CHAPTER 13

# The Many Faces of Gluten Intolerance

SUPPOSING A PERSON found a bakery providing whole grain organic rye bread, started consuming several slices a day and got diarrhea, constipation, bloating, fatigue, a rash consisting of tiny fluid-filled blisters, pallor, sleep disturbance, or just about any other symptom you could name? That individual might be one out of every hundred or so people who is sensitive to gluten: a protein in rye, wheat, barley and some other plant seeds that does not agree with people in a typically allergic way. It is not quite a peptide problem as described in chapter 10, and it is not limited to celiac disease, which is the diagnosis most often associated with gluten intolerance. Professor Luigi Greco of the Department of Pediatrics, University of Naples points out[47] that celiac disease, as it was known on the pediatric wards of European and American hospitals a generation or two ago, has tended to disappear while more subtle expressions of gluten intolerance are on the rise. He estimates that as many as one percent of the general population of Europe and America may have—or carry a potential to develop—gluten intolerance.

The understandable medical need for standard definitions of disease may cause some confusion when it comes to any given person's attempts to define his or her own potential for a problem with gluten. Gastroenterologists define gluten intolerance by microscopic changes observed in the cells lining the small intestine. An endoscope tube passed through the mouth, esophagus, stomach and upper part of the small intestine can be used to view the affected area. A biopsy can be taken to be examined microscopically for changes in the appearance of the finger-like projections that constitute the velvety surface of the intestine. The diagnosis of celiac disease may be made if the nap of this tissue is lost so that it becomes smooth and radically reduced in total surface area with the disappearance of all the finger-like projections. There are some individuals who have such changes in their small intestine and who are relatively symptom-free, and there are others who have a form of intolerance to gluten to which another name should apply because it causes symptoms without changes in the intestinal lining. Dr. Greco, however, is referring to the strict definition of gluten intolerance when he cites[48,49] a prevalence of gluten intolerance that should attract the attention of any person trying to sort out the possible causes of chronic health problems, especially, but not exclusively, if there are accompanying intestinal complaints. During my own efforts to understand the broad scope of the gluten problem I have been afflicted at times by the commonest cause of error among doctors: being blinded by the obvious.

The most dangerous circumstance that can arise when a patient presents with a complaint occurs when a ready explanation is immediately found. If a doctor reads an X-ray and finds an obvious abnormality, the chance of missing another finding that is more subtle and perhaps much more important to the patient's health becomes much higher than if the first distracting abnormality had not been there. Take Mr. Atlas, for example. He came to see me for a chronic problem with his bowels, and right away I found an intestinal parasite that seemed to be reason enough for bowel troubles. Treatment of the parasite, however, yielded only partial results. It took a long time and several repeated stool examinations before I realized that perhaps he had, so to speak, been sitting on two tacks, of which only one had been removed. Before his illness he had been a heavyweight boxer, and then a successful corporate attorney for whom a weight loss of 30 pounds was unwelcome, especially because he worked in an environment in which people tend to throw their weight around. Like all of us he wanted to stay in control and was understandably distressed as his authority over his own bowel waned. He found it humiliating to be summoned by it to the men's room in the middle of a high-level conference. He shared my initial relief at finding the parasite. He continued to complain of a symptom he had reported from the beginning, which I had failed to understand. He called it dry stools. I took this to mean the natural consequence of constipation in which the content of the lower intestine languishes as the body is bent on conserving water and the stool becomes hard. When we finally explored the details of this complaint, there turned out to be a difference between what he called dry and what I thought of as dry. I would have called it sticky. He had a difficult time cleaning himself after having a bowel movement.

Wheat is sticky. If you will forgive the sudden transition, I would like to point out that the paste most of us used (and ate) in kindergarten was made of wheat. The cultivation of wheat from its beginnings more than 9,000 years ago eventually gave rise to varieties of wheat that became numerous with early efforts to improve certain characteristics (such as more seeds per head of grain) and then diminished as a particular feature of wheat made it useful for making bread and pasta: stickiness. The adhesive qualities of gluten enable us to make a dough in which tiny bubbles can be formed by the "exhaled" carbon dioxide of the germs we use to leaven bread (usually yeast, but *lactobacillus* in the case of the Finnish rye bread mentioned earlier).* Leavening bread not only increases the stickiness of the dough, but liberates mineral nutrients to make it more nutritious. Needless to say, the refinement of flour that removes most of the minerals, vitamins and other important nutrients, including fiber, takes away the benefits derived from leavening.

When I realized that Mr. Atlas's stool was excessively sticky, I

---

* Baking soda is sodium bicarbonate and baking powder contains baking soda as well as another effervescent substance, potassium bitartrate. Both baking soda and baking powder form bubbles in batter or dough by the direct release of carbon dioxide when heated in the oven.

hazarded the guess that the stickiness could be from undigested gluten or products of the "leavening" of his dietary gluten by his intestinal germs. I performed a reasonably reliable blood test for detecting
antibodies that are markers for gluten sensitivity and only one was
abnormal. I took that as reason enough to ask him to forge ahead
with a gluten-free diet, which he was extremely reluctant to do. His
job entails numerous meetings where food, especially sandwiches, is
consumed. Moreover, his work milieu fosters individuals who value
toughness and skepticism. Few subjects arouse public skepticism
more than the claim "I can't eat it." People take being sensitive to
shellfish or strawberries without much objection, but having to
avoid the "staff of life" seems quite preposterous to some people.
Besides, if a person is sensitive to gluten, the quantities that may
cause symptoms may be so small that many prepared foods may
contain troublesome ingredients. Nothing is quite as disagreeable as
asking someone to avoid common foods, yet few medical practices
yield a more miraculous result when you hit the bull's eye. Mr. Atlas
hit it. Within days of going off wheat his bowel symptoms and his
annoyance with the diet evaporated.

## FOOD SENSITIVITIES AND THE DOMINO EFFECT

Gluten intolerance raises a special, but not entirely unique, relationship between intestinal function and sensitivities that appear to exist
with respect to food intolerance in general. A cycle of events can
occur in which the food sensitivity alters the function of the intestine
in ways that magnify the risk for acquiring more sensitivities. Another case will illustrate my point. I have known Seth Hammer for
20 years as a friend and building contractor as well as a person who
sought my medical advice on certain occasions. Some years ago he
asked me to investigate the possible factors that could have predis-
posed him to a stroke-like episode he suffered when he was in his
late 20s. That spell was somewhere in the gray zone between a severe migraine, which can be accompanied by neurologic deficits, and
a cerebrovascular accident in which some part of the brain is de-
prived of blood because of a clot or broken blood vessel. He recov-

ered from the previous attack and was not subject to migraine but lived in fear of another episode. Tests of his blood vessels at the time of his initial episode revealed no abnormalities, and the remainder of a complete neurologic evaluation was equally reassuring. When he asked me about it a few years later he was quite free of symptoms and I could not come up with a better approach than that recommended by the specialists he had seen before: it will probably not recur, so just relax and hope for the best. Last year it did recur. He found himself reading and not comprehending the words. He went to work and was able to do some intricate manual tasks but when attending a conference he could neither understand much of what was going on nor articulate beyond a few stray words. He developed a severe headache and does not remember anything that happened during his brief hospitalization. A complete neurologic evaluation was carried out and did not reveal a stroke, and he was signed out as a transient ischemic attack or TIA. Tests were completed to rule out some systemic illness such as lupus and they were all normal.

Seth came to see me a month or so later with the same question he had asked before, now intensified for obvious reasons. He is very healthy and able to run in marathons. He complained only of frequent dull headaches without any migrainous components (such as one-sidedness, visual symptoms, nausea and vomiting, or localized muscle weakness) and daytime somnolence to the point of falling asleep while reading stories to his daughter. He usually awakened several times during the night, woke up before his 5 a.m. alarm and did not feel refreshed by sleep.

Among the tests I carried out on him was an evaluation for food allergies as done by a blood test looking for antibodies. I was in the midst of designing the third phase of a research project involving testing for antibodies to foods of the IgG class. Antibodies are classified according to their size and shape, which correspond to different aspects of the immune response. Although the different roles of the type G, A, M, E and D antibodies are not completely understood, IgG testing is considered valid for gluten,[50,51] milk[52-54] and certain other substances.[55] Many physicians believe that only IgE is a marker for food allergy. I do not think that any particular antibody can account for the immune system's attitude toward a particular substance at any particular time. As I explained earlier it seems likely that the immune recognition system, like conscious perceptions, is orchestrated in flexible and subtle ways depending on the situation at hand. It is unreasonable to insist that any one mechanism, such as IgE, for example, is the sole reliable mediator of a whole class of immunological experiences. I do not think IgG is the only mediator of delayed food reactions. However there is abundant evidence that it is a clinically reliable marker for such reactions, provided there was analytical competence in the laboratory.

## MORE ON IgG-REACTIVE FOODS

The two pilot studies I have carried out so far have shown a high degree of statistical significance in the differences in symptom relief found when comparing matched groups of patients who avoided either IgG-reactive foods or were put on a placebo diet in an experiment in which the subjects did not know whether or not the foods they avoided were the ones that showed positive on their blood tests. I asked Seth to have a blood test as well as a functional test of his intestine that could be repeated after he avoided the foods that showed up as reactive on his blood test. If the intestinal test changed when he avoided certain foods, it would lend credence to the connection between his change in diet and any possible change in his symptoms. If his intestinal test and his symptoms both changed it would lend credence to the possibility that food sensitivity was a factor in his migraine-like attacks. Migraine is often caused by food sensitivity.[56-63] I thought food sensitivity should be considered in Seth's case even though the timing of his attacks was not at all suggestive of a food allergy pattern. Food allergy symptoms are often cyclic as the immune system engages in its feedback mechanisms that modulate its responses to stimuli. The response may build up to periodic crises that come at intervals that appear to have nothing to do with the calendar, menstrual or seasonal cycles or personal habits.

On the next page are Seth's results from his food allergy test. The foods followed by a number in parenthesis were reactive, and the others were nonreactive. The strength of the reaction is indicated by the number in parenthesis with +1 being the weakest and +4 being the strongest reaction.

Alfalfa
Almond
Apple
Apricot
Asparagus
Banana
Barley
**Bean, green (+1)**
**Bean, kidney (+1)**
Bean, pinto
**Bean, wax (+1)**
Beef
Blueberry
Broccoli
Brussels sprouts
Cabbage
Cantaloupe
Carrot
Cauliflower
Celery
Cheese
Cherry
Chicken
**Chili pepper (+1)**
Cinnamon

Clam
Clove
Cocoa-Chocolate
Cod
Coffee
Corn
Crab
Cucumber
**Egg (+1)**
Eggplant
Endive
Flounder
Garlic
Ginger
Grape
Grapefruit
**Haddock (+2)**
Halibut
Lamb
Lemon
Lettuce
Lime
Lobster
**Milk, cow's (+1)**
Mung bean
**Mushroom (+1)**

Mustard
Nutmeg
Oat
Olive
Onion
Orange
Oregano
Oyster
Parsley
Pea
Peach
Peanut
Pear
Pepper, black
Pepper, green
Pepper white
Pineapple
Plum
Pork
Potato, sweet
Potato white
**Radish (+2)**
Rice
**Rye (+1)**
Sage

Safflower
Salmon
Scallops
**Sesame (+3)**
Shrimp
Snapper
Sole
Soybean
Spinach
Strawberry
Sugar, cane
Sunflower
Tangerine
Tea
Tomato
Trout
Tuna
Turkey
Vanilla
Watermelon
Wheat
Whitefish
Yam
**Yeast, baker's (+1)**
**Yeast, brewer's (+1)**
Zucchini

The total number of IgG sensitivity reactions was 13 out of the 102 foods tested. That is about average for allergic people. I felt that it was consistent with Seth having allergy problems, but the degree of reactivity was not high. I did not take this too seriously because the plan was simple enough: Seth was to avoid all the reactive foods for a month and see how he felt while checking if anything changed in his intestinal permeability test.

## Testing for Intestinal Leaks

Of all the functions of the intestine, the most basic one is keeping the food and fecal stream separate from the bloodstream. Considering that the intestinal membrane is about the thickness of an eyelid, it is remarkable that this cavity with its toxic contents can be so close to the bloodstream without causing more trouble. Whenever there is trouble in the intestine, a leak of substances into the bloodstream is one of the first consequences. In the laboratory this leak is measured by a simple test in which, in Seth's case, for example, he was asked to drink a glass of a beverage containing two kinds of sugar. Neither one is used by our body, but one, mannitol, is absorbed to some degree into the bloodstream whence it passes unchanged into the urine via the kidneys. In the six hours following ingestion of the mannitol, the 5 to 25 percent that is absorbed under normal conditions appears in the urine. Another sugar, lactulose, passes unchanged into the stools and only a very small fraction (less than 8 parts in a thousand) is normally absorbed and then excreted in the urine. The amount of each sugar gives an idea of whether there is a problem with poor absorption of what should be absorbed or abnormal leakiness of substances that ought not to be absorbed. I have used this test for years in my practice and find it to be one of the most sensitive and useful tests of intestinal function. It is not a test that makes a diagnosis of a particular disease, but one that measures a function that can go wrong and should be corrected no matter what disease is in the patient's picture. Let us look at Seth's results. He repeated the permeability test twice, once each on two consecutive days because of a misunderstanding that turned out to be very fortunate. His first test was so abnormal that I would have thought it to be a rare laboratory error. It was not. Here are both test results:

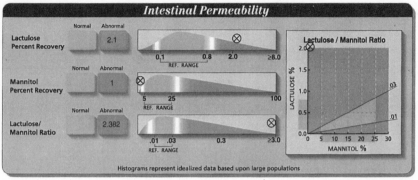

FIGURE 1

**Seth's First Permeability Test**

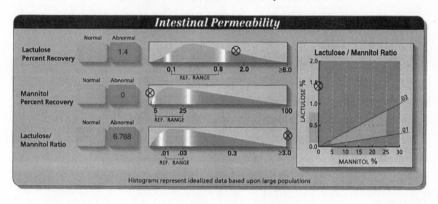

FIGURE 2

**Seth's Second Permeability Test**

The second test showed comparable abnormalities. If you look at the two figures you will see that Seth's absorption of lactulose, as shown by its recovery from his urine, was very high in both tests. It should have fallen in the light gray reference range of 0.3–0.8 percent and instead it was greater than 2 percent on the first test and 1.4 percent on the second test. His mannitol, on the other hand, was extremely low: 1 percent and 0 on the two tests. It is intriguing that such a profound abnormality of intestinal function existed in a person who had no digestive symptoms.

Seth embarked on his diet, avoiding the reactive foods. Here are my notes from an office visit after Seth returned for a follow-up visit about two months later:

> Going off the foods was associated with a spectacular change in gut permeability. During the diet headache and drowsiness disappeared and since going back on the avoided foods the afternoon and evening fatigue (which was intensified after the TIA) reappeared. The quality of sleep was markedly changed: for many months before going on the diet, sleep was interrupted just to awaken or to urinate. Normally alarm is set for 5 a.m. and he was always awake before the alarm. After three to four days on the diet he did not awaken during the night, did not awaken before the alarm and actually slept through the alarm. After restarting eggs he had extreme fatigue and poor sleep quality; after second egg exposure he had the same. On May 18, he had a cruller, then a bagel and both times fatigue and early wakening occurred. That (yeast) reaction was extreme. On May 24 he had 2 pieces of pizza. By 7:30 that evening he was passed out on the couch. Had to go to bed at 9:30. Quality of sleep was average. Awakened before the alarm on May 27, he had had eggs in the morning. Reaction was not as great as before. Subsequently had pasta, cheese, mushroom, egg, milk and since then has not felt right.

On the next page are the results of his permeability test after four weeks on the diet. Notice that his lactulose and mannitol absorption became completely normal so that the graphic representation of their relationship shows up on the right side of the diagram as the circled x within the normal triangular zone.

## Some Conclusions

Seth's case illustrates the following key points:

1. The intestine and its function are common sources of problems even when digestive symptoms are absent.

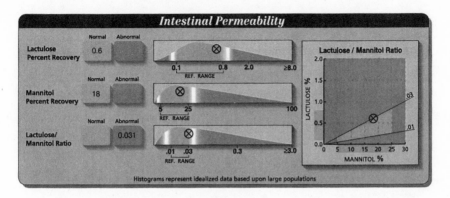

FIGURE 3

**Seth's Permeability Test After Avoiding IgG Reactive Foods**

2. Symptoms are sometimes related to a complex interconnectedness of factors and do not follow simple cause-and-effect relationships. The egg and a few of the other problem foods did not cause his symptoms in the same sense as stubbing the toe causes its pain or catching a virus causes chicken pox. The foods caused alterations in intestinal permeability, which allowed more unwanted substances to enter his bloodstream, which caused an overload of his detoxication systems (which I was able to document by other lab tests), which caused alterations in his chemistry which resulted in his symptoms and perhaps lowered his threshold for having a stroke-like migraine in ways that we cannot completely understand.

3. Relatively minor symptoms can be important clues to success. Even if we did not have the laboratory evidence to suggest that Seth's health changed dramatically when he avoided certain foods, his symptoms gave both him and me a strong impression that the benefits he achieved apply to his risk of TIA.

4. There is an effort to find as many things wrong as can be reasonably and reliably identified. I take steps to correct each one without always being able to estimate its contribution to the overall problem. Of all the aspects of the systems approach to medicine, this is the one that at first seems most

uncomfortable to those of us with a traditional training that has imbued us with a respect for parsimony. "The physician who treats least treats best" is an admonition with a strong pull. Its attraction is especially forceful in a medical tradition in which treatment usually carries a significant inherent danger. The systems approach usually employs remedies that are not very dangerous, are aimed at restoring balance and often demand several remedies given together. To not find and fix as many sources of imbalance as can be found seems negligent.

5. The patient and the doctor share a comfort with speculation and uncertainty. If I had diagnosed Seth's daily headaches as tension headaches and given him a prescription, he and I could have been certain, in a way, that it was the "right treatment." But that is not why he came to see me. He wanted to embark on a course that he and I knew might not fetch any answers but which followed a certain logic that he understood from our previous consultations. I will present the logic in the next chapter.

# CHAPTER 14

# The Map:

## A Guide to Thoroughness in Approaching Health Problems

USING THE MAP on page 125 as a tool for understanding health problems is not much different from the kind of thinking you would do if the Swedish ivy plant on your window sill failed to thrive. The following two questions would precede any attempt on your part to make a diagnosis, in the sense of giving a name to the ivy's condition beyond "not doing well," "wilting," or "withering." You would first consider whether you failed to give the plant something it requires to flourish and then wonder if the plant might be exposed to something that did not agree with it. If you know anything at all about horticulture, you would understand that these two questions are interconnected. If a plant is stressed by pests, germs or toxins, it may require more nutrients; if it is undernourished it may be more susceptible to the effects of pests, germs or toxins. Human beings are more complex than Swedish ivies in that we need a greater variety of nutrients and are subject to a greater variety of germs and toxins, but the most important difference between us and ivies is that there is a greater variety among us than there is among Swedish ivies.

The pioneer nutritional biochemist, Roger Williams,[64] pointed to a 200-fold difference in calcium requirements among different healthy human subjects. Recent research in the toxicity of mercury has revealed sensitivities to mercury that vary as much as a million-fold from one individual to another.[65,66] Why is it that we are all so unique? I am privileged to have as a friend Charles Remington, Ph.D., Emeritus Professor of Biology at Yale, one of the world's foremost scholars in the field of insects and evolutionary biology. During butterfly watching and pleasant evenings in front of the fire sharing his vast knowledge of biology, he has explained to me that individuals in a species tend to vary more if their habitat has been disturbed. For example, if you study all the creatures in a certain area and observe variations in color, size and other characteristics of individual members of a given species of bird, insect or mammal they will resemble one another closely if they have all been living in the same undisturbed habitat for many generations. Then, if there is a major disruption caused by fire, flood, deforestation or other calamity, the species who remain to repopulate the territory will go through an extended period in which they will show marked diversity among individuals until the environment achieves a new stability.

## TREATING THE INDIVIDUAL—*NOT* A DIAGNOSTIC CATEGORY

We human beings are quite consciously aware that each of us is different from everyone else. I don't think that the notion of our individual uniqueness is a conceit. It is firmly based on biology and probably is enhanced by the fact that our habitat has changed as much as that of any creature during the last few thousand years of migration, the establishment of agriculture and the addition of thousands of new chemicals to the human environment. However, it is easier to group people to avoid the complexity of thinking about and treating each person as an individual. Supposing I were to fill out an insurance form for Seth Hammer and report that he has Seth Hammer's disease and that I am giving him the Seth Hammer treatment. The map that I will show you in this chapter makes the purpose of thinking about individuals much clearer, but it does not help with insurance forms. It has been 40 years since Roger Williams' research and writing introduced a new paradigm for medicine backed by solid scientific research. It is not a lack of science that has retarded the blossoming of a medical practice focused more on individuality. It has more to do with the inertia of a medical hierarchy that yields slowly to change and the strong investment of various levels of the hierarchy in treating diseases, not individuals.

It is not just that doctors think in terms of diseases but that a whole structure of fund raising, allocation of resources for research, reimbursement for medical care, medical education and specialization is based on the idea that diseases exist in nature as fixed entities. We do not need to give up the idea of diseases nor yield to the understanding that our picture of disease is a transient artifact of our limited ways of seeing groups of individuals. We can begin to improve on our system for taking care of individuals, with or without having a name for their disorder, by applying a simple strategy for problem solving. I invite you to consider such a way of thinking about any chronic complaint that you may develop, whether your chronic symptoms fall neatly into a diagnostic category or whether your symptoms cannot quite be summed up under a given disease name. I will return to the origins of disease names and classifications in chapter 17.

## THE INDIVIDUAL APPROACH

If we take the strategy for treating Swedish ivy and apply it to Seth or to Sylvia Franco or to any person, a logical question flows from each of the first two questions.

1. What kinds of things does this person need to get in order to thrive?
2. What kinds of things does this person need to avoid in order to thrive?

By current knowledge the kinds of things a person needs in order to thrive are vitamins, minerals, fatty acids, amino acids, accessory nutritional factors, light, healthy rhythms (see chapter 16) and to love and be loved. When I first began thinking along the lines of the map, I was intimidated by my lack of knowledge of nutritional biochemistry and the environmental factors associated with allergy and toxicity. It seemed to me that the disease-oriented approach, which I had mastered to a certain extent, was a more comfortable domain in which to think about problems. Soon, however, I realized that there is an elegant simplicity to the map that is governed by the realities of biochemistry and of our environment: there are only so many nutrients and accessory nutritional factors and there are only so many foods, inhalants and toxins to which a person can be exposed.

By current knowledge the kinds of things a person needs to avoid in order to thrive are allergens, which are things that, in small amounts, bother some people more than others; and toxins, which also vary in their capacity to bother a given person, but are more uniformly harmful. Just about any substance can act as an allergen. Therefore it is helpful to break the possibilities into categories in order to make the prospects less overwhelming. Those categories are food, pollen, dust, animal dander, chemicals, mold and other microorganisms. To be considered as a possible cause of problems a substance has to be in either one of the two ways each of us divides the universe: our insides or our outsides. That may seem like an unnecessarily naïve point, but it goes to the question of whether the strategy is thorough. It is reassuring to think that one's view of possibilities is all-encompassing and that nothing is overlooked before one begins to whittle them down through a process of elimination.

When it comes to toxins, the possibilities are: elementary substances such as lead, mercury and aluminum; compounds produced by living creatures including ourselves and our germs; and synthetic compounds, most of which are products of petrochemicals which in turn come from seriously decayed oil that was once produced by living creatures. Radiation of various kinds is potentially toxic as well.

## The Map and How It Is Used

### Map for a Thorough Approach to Health Problems

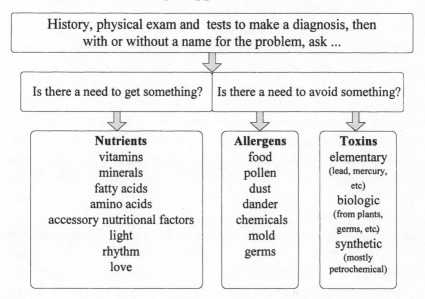

Here is the map with an emphasis on the point that this strategy is not a substitute for the standard medical approach that includes taking a history, doing a complete physical exam and conducting laboratory tests to make a diagnosis with special attention to thinking of all the worst things that could be wrong. The map serves as a guide whether my patient has a *definitive* diagnosis such as diabetes, Crohn's disease or psoriasis; a *descriptive* diagnosis such as hyperactivity, depression or tinnitus; or a collection of symptoms that match no diagnostic category. It may be relatively easy to accept that if symptoms match no diagnostic category, then the map may serve as a guide to finding out what is wrong. It may be difficult to understand how the map can be helpful for people who already have a diagnosis. Having a diagnosis implies that the condition is more or less understood. That is just the problem. Having a label for a problem may lead to the conclusion that all symptoms are "caused by"

the diagnosis. Further thinking tends to stop more easily than if the basic question of what is wrong is left open without a label. Remember that the most common mistakes that we doctors make are the result of finding one thing wrong and being lulled into a relaxed frame of mind about further detective work. I have already referred to this as being "blinded by the obvious."

In explaining this map to patients I recruit their participation in the diagnostic process. Even after patients have filled out a 20-page questionnaire and written a chronology of their major life events, illnesses, operations, schooling, jobs, losses and successes, additional clues emerge when reviewing this strategy. For example, a woman recovering from surgery and chemotherapy for her metastatic breast cancer once consulted me wondering what she might do to maximize her chances of staying well. Her history seemed quite lacking in risk factors, and her initial biochemical and immunologic evaluation was surprisingly free of the kinds of abnormalities I would have expected. In reviewing the situation with her I repeated my recitation of the map, covering each item in the above diagram as I described its logic. When I mentioned toxins she asked if there could be any significance to the fact that her home had a strange odor. The house was built of natural cedar, and a preservative, pentachlorophenol, was then applied to all the interior and exterior surfaces. The odor was quite like cedar and was at its strongest in certain interior spaces, particularly a nook where their dog, now dead of cancer, had slept. I referred her to my associate, Dr. Bob McLellan, a specialist in occupational health. Her tests revealed a level of pentachlorophenol in her urine that was substantially above the maximum permitted in workers in a pentachlorophenol factory. During the ensuing months her home was treated to seal in the toxin so that it could neither be touched nor inhaled, and she and her husband were given supplements to support their detoxification chemistry. She remains well today and is content to be uncertain whether her long-term exposure to a chemical toxin had a role in her susceptibility to cancer. Doubts about the connection never made it seem reasonable to leave the situation alone.

The map is not a menu for doing lab tests. Most of the factors listed can be evaluated with lab tests, but the map is simply a guide to a complete list of questions beginning with the word "could." "Could this person have a magnesium deficiency or a special need for magnesium that contributes to his or her problem? Could this person have accumulated an unhealthy amount of aluminum that is contributing to his or her problem?" The literature on the incidence of deficiencies or special nutritional needs and the prevalence of toxins in our environment provides ample scientific backing to the legitimacy of at least posing the question. It is beyond the scope of this book to explore all of the laboratory tests that cover each consideration in the map. The next chapter will describe tests that constitute the highest priorities with respect to evaluating the chemistry of detoxification.

## HOW PEOPLE BECOME SENSITIVE

The part of the map that refers to allergies carries another implied question that arises when sensitivity is a factor to be considered. The question is, "If this person is sensitive to one or more substances that contribute to his or her illness, then how did he or she become sensitive?" Why are people sensitive anyway? We know what sensitivity is: it is a reaction to something that does not bother most people at all or at least not to the same extent. It can be called allergy, hypersensitivity or intolerance without much precision in distinguishing among those terms. We know how to recognize it and I will share with you some ideas I have about how people become sensitive, but we really do not know precisely what changes when a person goes from having a normal tolerance for a food, pollen, animal dander, chemical, mold or germ to having an intolerance. I have mentioned certain lab tests that are helpful, but even if I were able to peer anywhere into a person's cellular makeup, down to the level of molecules and up to the level of organization of a person's electromagnetic fields, I would not know where to look for the thing that has changed from the time before he or she became sensitive to milk, eggs, strawberries, mold or perfume. We know that the capacity to become sensitized is a capacity shared by the nervous system and the immune system, which provides further evidence for their unity. We know the kinds of cells that are involved in sensitivity in each case, but we do not understand the changes in those cells that account for their change in "attitude." Without knowing exactly where sensitivity is, it is still possible to find reasons why people become sensitive.

I began accumulating the following list from listening to the stories of patients who came to see me with problems of sensitivity to many things, sometimes so many things that controlling their diet and environment seemed a fairly unworkable treatment compared to finding the sensitivity's basis and repairing that. The list provides a helpful orientation to considering ways to evaluate a person's detoxification chemistry, which I will cover in the next chapter.

**1. Something is out of balance.** If am standing on one foot and you push me over with your thumb, I could conclude that I am thumb-sensitive and need to stay away from thumbs. Now if I put both feet on the ground I regain my balance and I am no longer so sensitive to the effect of your thumb. In the same way a toddler with eczema may itch all over and keep himself up half the night scratching because of sensitivities to foods, fabrics, dust or other factors that cannot easily be determined. He just seems sensitive to everything. Then, for example, if a zinc deficiency is found and his balance is restored with respect to zinc, his sensitivity will diminish.

**2. Something is wrong with digestion.** If the destructive forces of digestion are lacking and more than normal quantities of food substances escape being stripped of the antigenicity by which they are able to provoke allergic reactions, then it is the fault of digestion, not the immune system. I realize that I am being unfaithful to the whole cyberhealth concept by starting to cast blame on this or that system. However, once allergy is provoked by poor digestion, digestion may be the victim of allergy as was true in Seth's case. So it goes round and round in a circle. Circular effects are the rule.

Magnesium deficiency provides another example. A person under stress tends to lose excess magnesium as part of the response to stress. A magnesium deficit then creates the setting for less resistance to stress. The question is not so much which part of the circle is to blame, but which is the most practical place to intervene to break the cycle. If a person is sensitive to most foods and has very poor stomach acid secretion or a failure to produce good bile or other digestive juices, then supporting those functions with supplements makes more sense than severe dietary restriction. I have already described permeability problems as being mutually linked with sensitivities.

**3. Infection.** If the immune system has to get up every day and fight germs it is not surprising that it may become cranky and overly reactive to environmental stimuli. I think that "hypervigilant" is a good term for describing the posture of the immune system that has taken on an increased reactivity to many kinds of substances. Such a posture is part of a state of immune activation that is common in individuals with many illnesses including autoimmune conditions, chronic fatigue immunodeficiency syndrome and childhood autism as well as generalized tendencies toward allergy. The place in the body where germs are least accessible to control by our various immune mechanisms is the intestinal tract, where parasites and the overgrowth of yeasts are the most common provokers of a hypervigilant immune system.

If I meet someone casually and he or she describes a relative's problem and says no more than that the person in question was quite well until a certain point when he or she became suddenly sensitive to all sorts of foods, chemicals or dust, my very first thought is that the person must have been on antibiotics in the interval before the onset of the state of hypersensitivity which was caused by a yeast problem. Virus infections are also capable of a tenacious chronicity, and the ones that have the greatest capacity for ongoing subtle mischief are Herpes simplex and Epstein-Barr virus.

**4. Chemical exposure.** An exposure to any potential allergen can sensitize a person if the exposure is intense or if it is accompanied by a high level of stress, even if the stress is not painful. When I joined the Peace Corps I had finished my six-month stint as an assistant resident in obstetrics and gynecology and suddenly found myself getting up early in California not to deliver babies but to play soccer with Peace Corps volunteers who were just out of college and in much better shape than I. Leaving my cat, car, house and belongings to be cared for by someone else for two years and traveling with my then wife and nine-month-old daughter across the country constituted stress. When I started having to get up at night to treat myself for asthma attacks I suspected that I was having some sort of emotional reaction to the Peace Corps. A vacationing friend of my wife's then returned to claim her cat who had been boarding with us, and my asthma disappeared. My severe cat allergy lingered and some years later I realized that my sensitization must have had something to do with the cat-stress combination, especially considering that I had had cats all along. Returning from Africa after two years I found myself unable to tolerate my old cat's presence!

If, instead of being exposed to a cat, I had moved into an environment that was contaminated with formaldehyde, pesticides or petroleum-derived chemicals from fuel oil to plastics, I might have not only overloaded my detoxication system's capacity to rid myself of my daily load of inhaled or ingested material, but something more insidious could have happened: the engendering of a global state of sensitivity to "all" chemicals. Such a state stretches scientific credulity. First of all there has been a long-standing belief in the field of allergy that only fairly large molecules can provoke an allergic response and most of the substances we informally group under the heading "chemicals" are small molecules. Moreover, they are a diverse group, and allergy is understood to be quite specific. Finally, the symptoms reported by victims of chemical sensitization are often cerebral and subjective in nature, inviting the reproach that "it is all in your head." Individuals who suffer from chemical sensitivity often find themselves in a surprisingly adversarial medical setting in which physicians state firmly that they "do not believe in" chemical sensitivity and cite the finding of emotional disorders in chemically sensitive patients[67] as evidence that there is no physiologic basis for the problem, which therefore must be a state of malingering or psychosis. A person who has become chemically sensitized enters a much more polarized medical setting than someone who has been sensitized to cats, and should be forewarned of encounters with physicians who hold strong positions that whatever is wrong with such patients is "not real."

The controversy over chemical sensitization, sometimes referred to as multiple chemical sensitivity or MCS, has been explored thoroughly in Canada, where the Ministries of Health are obliged to take definite positions regarding the eligibility of patients for benefits and physicians for reimbursement in connection with MCS. The report of the Environmental Hypersensitivities Workshop of the Ministry of Health in Ottawa states in its executive summary:

> Given its clinical prominence and the attendant socioeconomic costs, multiple chemical sensitivities (MCS) is worthy of scientific study. In the meantime, however, the patient should not be caught in the medical debate and denied social benefits. Benefits should be based on defined functional disabilities, not on the medical label. Ministries of Health should be responsible for ensuring that there is no discrimination against patients by insurance companies in regard to coverage for medical-related expenses.

The MCS controversy has been investigated by the State of New Jersey, which commissioned a study by Nicholas Ashford, Ph.D., J.D. and Claudia Miller M.D.[68] Ashford and Miller provide detailed support for the concept of chemical sensitivity. The United States Department of Housing and Urban Development has adopted a clear, legally supported policy recognizing chemical sensitivity as a disability requiring reasonable accommodations by landlords.[69] The Social Security Administration recognizes MCS as a disabling condition in the sense that a person may have the physical capacity to perform work, but if unavoidable environmental exposures cause debilitating symptoms, a disability exists.[70]

The concept of sensitizing potential was first championed by the late Dr. Theron Randolph, who became the father of an ecologic approach to medicine and teacher of many of us who found ourselves in the practice of various specialties, knowing a great deal about our patient's innards and very little about their "outards," that is, the physical and chemical environment with which their chemistry interacted. Although Dr. Randolph's work coincided in the 1960s with the general awakening to the realities of chemical pollution as a general phenomenon, the medical profession's focus on disease left it poorly prepared to accept the very individual nature of chemical sensitivity and slow to accept the idea that a patient's toxic burden might constitute a clinical priority no matter what his or her disease may be.

Dr. William Rea is the Randolph disciple who has done more than anyone to bring a passionate and scholarly energy to the study and treatment of problems of chemical sensitization and chemical poisoning. His multivolume treatise, *Chemical Sensitivity*,[71] presents the most comprehensive review of the subject. Dr. Sherry Rogers' books[72] provide another rich resource of information about chemical sensitivity.

**5. Adrenal insufficiency.** Here is a story that exemplifies a common finding in sensitive individuals. Abigail Stockwell was at the Sleigh House restaurant one evening in 1980 when an obstructed flue filled the place with gas fumes. She was among dozens of patrons who were treated in the emergency room for a variety of symptoms from fainting, nausea and headache to numbness and tingling. One of the puzzling things about chemical exposures is the great variety of symptoms that can be produced in different individuals from an essentially identical exposure. Before that exposure she was well except for a childhood history of eczema. After it she was troubled by fatigue, nausea, a peculiar scratching pain in her head, difficulty concentrating and depression. Such symptoms would recur particularly following exposure to a variety of petroleum-based products. Pumping her own gasoline could make her sick for a couple of days. She was bothered by certain foods as well as by pollen, dust and molds. When I first interviewed her I thought that she was sensitized by her initial exposure to gas fumes and that her recovery would be more difficult to achieve than it would be for someone with sensitivities limited to foods or mold. I asked her about symptoms of fatigue, feeling cold, recurring infection, low blood pressure, poor modulation of blood sugar, salt craving, acne and other hormonal symptoms such as excessive facial or body hair or loss of scalp hair. These are all indicators of a common condition (about one in 100 people) called congenital adrenal hyperplasia or CAH. The only symptoms she reported from the list were hair loss, fatigue and feeling cold in the evening. I did not think that she was a very good candidate for CAH. After failed attempts to treat her by removing mold from her diet and killing yeasts in her intestines, I did a simple test to rule out CAH which involved a trial of treatment while monitoring her symptoms with a key lab test before and after the trial. Here is the information I gave her and the instructions for the brief test treatment.

### Low-dose hydrocortisone therapy

Hydrocortisone is the normal product of your adrenal gland. It is the main hormone among a whole family called steroid hormones. Some people fail to produce enough hydrocortisone to provide for their body's needs. Like people with low thyroid function, such people benefit from taking hormone pills to make up for what their body fails to produce each day. The average daily production of hydrocortisone in your body is about 30 to 40 mg. If you have adrenal insufficiency (low adrenal function) you may be producing only 15 to 25 mg daily and consequently may feel cold and tired, have many sensitivities, low blood pressure and salt craving. By supplementing your low production with, say, 5 to 20 mg of hydrocortisone your body's supply becomes normal and symptoms should promptly disappear.

The big misunderstanding that occurs with regard to this treatment comes from the use of high-dose cortisone or cortisone-like medicines (prednisone, Medrol, etc.). With high-dose treatment, doses way in excess of your body's needs are given and have a serious drug effect plus many side effects: high blood pressure, weight gain (usually with a characteristic central distribution and a moon face), immune suppression with a tendency toward fungus infections, diabetes, stomach ulcers and so on. These potential side effects have nothing to do with what could happen with low-dose hydrocortisone treatment which cannot give your body significantly more than your body needs. Even if your production of hydrocortisone is already normal, the extra 5 to 20 mg hardly ever makes a noticeable difference. High-dose treatment employs amounts of cortisone or cortisone-like drugs (prednisone) equivalent to at least several times your body's daily output, that is, 60 to 300 mg of hydrocortisone per day.

So, if a friend says, "Oh my God, you're not taking cortisone, are you? That stuff is so dangerous, my mother took it and it gave her ulcers and she gained weight!" please reassure yourself and your friend that you are using this medicine in a totally different and safe way. Can tests be done before actually taking this treatment to determine if it is really needed before trying it? Yes, but . . . The tests are very good at picking up people with bad adrenal insufficiency, but they can miss people who need low-dose hydrocortisone treatment. I have done the tests in dozens of people and have decided that the best first test is a clinical trial of hydrocortisone. It is without risk and takes less time and trouble than the tests. If you fail to feel better from taking the hydrocortisone, then you don't need the test. If you feel much better, so that it appears that you needed the hydrocortisone, then a test can be done later to confirm the diagnosis, if that seems appropriate. Note that low-dose hydrocortisone is used to treat people with mild adrenal insufficiency in whom the symptoms of underproduction of hydrocortisone come out as an overproduction of "male" type hormones that lead in women to scalp hair loss, excessive hair growth, and other hormonal abnormalities.[73]

**Dosage schedule**

Take a dose of 2.5 mg daily (any time, preferably not with food) for 3 to 4 days. See how it feels. Then increase to 1 dose of 2.5 mg twice daily and see how it feels for 3 to 4 days. Then increase to 1 dose of 2.5 mg three times daily and see how it feels, working up to 1 dose of 2.5 mg four times daily after a few more days. Continue stepwise to a maximum of 20 mg daily (still divided into 4 doses). Don't worry if the pill doesn't break exactly in two, the precision of dosage is not critical. A few people who do not need the hydrocortisone may feel a little "too good" or have trouble with sleep or feel a little bloated and should reduce the dose to a level that does not produce any side effects. In such a case you should continue with the lower dose for the few weeks that it takes to see if symptoms are cleared. This diagnostic trial is free of risk and should give an answer to the question of mild adrenal insufficiency within three weeks. If there is no difference in such symptoms as feeling cold, tired, salt craving, low blood pressure, dizziness, acne, excessive hair growth, multiple sensitivities or other symptoms particular to your expression of adrenal insufficiency within a few weeks, discontinue the medication. . . . you do not have mild adrenal insufficiency and we will have to look for other causes of your problems! Remember that this is low-dose treatment and is very different from taking steroids in large amounts. Hydrocortisone is about five times less potent than prednisone, so the equivalent doses of prednisone that are used to treat allergic and other inflammatory diseases, say 40 mg daily, would be 200 mg of hydrocortisone.

Mrs. Stockwell became 50 percent better after the first few weeks of treatment when she had arrived at a dose of 2.5 mg of hydrocortisone 4 times daily. After that she went on to make a complete recovery and now can go about her business in New York City with only occasional symptoms when she encounters the exhaust of a diesel bus or someone wearing too much perfume in an elevator. As part of her initial evaluation I had done a study of her detoxification chemistry. I will describe it in the next chapter and show you how it became completely normal after she was treated. The normalization of her detoxification chemistry provides a good example of the interconnections among immune function, adrenal function and detoxification. It may turn out that after a few months of treatment she will no longer need her hydrocortisone.

Adrenal insufficiency can result from a congenital weakness in the biochemistry that forms hydrocortisone in the adrenal gland. In its extreme form it produces a masculinization of girl babies to the point that their clitoris and other external genitals are enlarged to a male appearance. Unless the condition is recognized immediately the associated imbalance in the regulation of body salts can precipitate a fatal crisis. At the very least, a delay in the proper assignment of gender can result in distress for everyone involved. Many people with adrenal insufficiency have a very mild form of the same condition. They do not have genital abnormalities but may show, after maturity, salt cravings, excess hair growth and acne as well as the other symptoms mentioned above. On the other hand, an unknown percentage of individuals with adrenal weakness acquire it from stress. This was first studied by Hans Selye, the famous physiologist whose studies of soldiers killed in battle clarified the relationship between the adrenal gland and stress. A certain number of the healthy 17- to 20-year-old young men who are found dead on a battlefield have no wounds to explain their death. At post mortem examination, the only abnormality found is an exceptional shrinkage of the adrenal glands. These and other studies conducted by Dr. Selye over many years gave rise to the whole modern concept of the relationship between stress and health. In a sense, my profession received the concept of stress with open arms but not so with the findings about the adrenal glands. The reasons for that turn of events are discussed in the monograph[73] by the endocrinologist William Jefferies. Considering Mrs. Stockwell's lack of long-term masculinizing symptoms and the sudden onset of her illness after a chemical exposure I think that her condition may be temporary so that in several months or a year she can come off the hormone support and find that her health and tests are normal.

**6. Invasive life events.** In the course of a two-hour initial visit patients with multiple sensitivities often refer to the unforgettable pain and anger of experiences suffered in childhood that were abusive, often in a very literally invasive way. This abuse need not always have been sexual; even certain medical procedures (such as a tonsillectomy performed in the kitchen, believe it or not) could easily be interpreted by a child as a violation accompanied by severe pain. For some the revelation of such stories had gone unspoken for many years. Especially in respect to sexual abuse, if feelings of anger and pain do not find their natural exit in speech they are more likely to burrow into a person's soul and do mischief that may be expressed more immunologically than psychologically on the surface. When such patients have pursued the appropriate psychological treatment, the immunologic aspects of their hypervigilance become much more responsive to treatment.

This may be the appropriate place to make the point that I do not think that health is concerned only with biochemistry and immunology. I have chosen those subjects for this book to clarify the central role of detoxification chemistry, but I do not mean to suggest that words and deeds and the feelings they engender cannot be toxic.

On the contrary, I believe that words and deeds have the greatest potential for harm and healing and that only when they are in the right balance can the biochemical and immunological treatments prevail. We live, however, in a culture with a high level of psychological awareness. If a person is feeling chronically sad without apparent reason, appropriate attempts to find a psychological reason or to alleviate symptoms temporarily with drugs should not fail to include a look for biochemical balance.

CHAPTER 15

# How Detoxification Works

RETURNING FROM LUNCH to my cottage I spotted a monarch butterfly boldly flitting and gliding on the July breeze across the meadow. I say boldly because the meadow is inhabited by birds who would gladly make a meal of any number of passing insects including most butterflies. Not, however, of a monarch, one of the most poisonous creatures to travel the meadows of North America where it migrates annually thousands of miles to and from its winter home in Mexico. Poisons in the monarch's milkweed meals during its caterpillar stages accumulate in its body, neither being detoxified nor cast off during the transformation from larval stages to the winged adult. The poisons are safely sequestered in the wings, the least metabolically active parts of the butterfly, so that they harm only whatever animal might attempt to eat it. Thus, the monarch carries poisons as its license to parade its beauty in public with little danger of being eaten. A bird who takes only one less-than-deadly taste of a monarch will remember its mistake six months later and refuse any such meal again.[74] The monarch, like many insects, takes advantage of the poisonous nature of its host plant. Except for certain mechanisms for spreading their seeds, plants, in general, do not want to be eaten. Consider the millions of different kinds of plants on earth and the relatively small number that we humans are able to eat, and then remember that even those are not completely free of toxins. To be a plant is to be toxic in some way as part of a mechanism, however attenuated in some species, of self-protection. I have often watched my goats eat. They browse in the fields and woods with a careful preference for certain leaves that they can sniff out with a gourmet's discrimination. Their menu is much more varied than mine, in which very few leaves are represented. The goats have germs high up in their digestive processes which not only digest cellulose but detoxify many of the substances in plants that could never be tolerated in animals that lack a rumen.

We humans have neither the front-end protection of a stomach full of cleaver germs or the downstream capability of sequestering toxins in our body, although we do have a minor talent for putting some toxic metals into our hair bound to the same sticky sulfur atoms that fasten the stranded molecules in position in each hair shaft. How then, do we deal with unwanted substances that get into us via our food, water and air? How can we measure not only how many toxins we have accumulated but, more important, how can we test the efficiency of our detoxification machinery, the biggest part of our biochemistry?

## DETOXIFICATION—A COSTLY PROCESS

Let me elaborate on the last point before returning to follow some sample toxins through the system. One of the main points of this book is that some of the most troublesome toxins are ones that look so much like friendly molecules that they escape detection until they have already done mischief by masquerading as invited participants in a key biochemical step. You might expect that there is a major distinction between the way the body handles these substances and the friendly ones they mimic and the way it handles recognizably unwanted molecules, such as lead or various plant toxins. I have already said in chapter 9 that reduced glutathione, one of the princely members of our family of detoxification chemicals, is *lost* from the body when a foreign chemical is detoxified while it is *recovered* from detoxification operations when the toxic substances are generated from our own chemistry. Otherwise everything in the body, all the molecules left over from the daily operations of the brain, bowels, blood, bones, muscles, skin and all the internal organs require the use of the same chemistry that is used for dealing with naturally occurring toxins as well as with the environmental pollutants that enter with our food, water and air. That is why cleansing the body of unwanted substances is the most costly metabolic activity in which our chemistry engages.

For a child, the cost of growth is also very high, but in adults, detoxification is the major molecule-making activity. That's right, *molecule making.* Detoxification in human beings mostly involves synthesis as opposed to degradation. Even detoxification jobs that look as if they are mostly breaking things down turn out, in the end, to involve costly steps in which new molecules are made just for the sake of safe disposal. Remember methylmalonic acid. It is the stuff that may pile up in the body's process of getting rid of the amino acid, valine. When the broken step I described in chapter 11 is working well, the object of the disassembly line I described is to take the amino group off of the amino acid so that what remains can burn clean in the citric acid cycle. But amino groups, removed from their amino acid or protein origins, turn into ammonia—the same strong poison that you recognize by its noxious odor. Ammonia cannot simply be allowed to go free inside your cells or in your blood. It is captured by alpha ketoglutarate (AKG), also mentioned in chapter 11, which becomes glutamate. Glutamate can take on another ammonia to become glutamine, which, in turn, delivers the unwanted ammonia to the single most expensive chemical department in the body, the urea cycle, where an elaborate process of handing off the ammonia is carried out with the final formation of urea which can safely pass through the kidneys and out of the body. The breaking down of each amino acid molecule eventually requires making a molecule. The making of molecules for detoxification requires the lion's share of all the energy we expend on making any kind of molecule every day.

We go about our daily chores without conscious attention to

the molecular details of our body's management of toxins, allergens and other waste, but if our sanitation department did make itself known to us—say by making a noise—it would drown out all the comparable noises of walking, thinking and talking. Imagine the machinery of detoxification, mostly in the liver, emitting an enormous grinding, groaning, gurgling sound that would dwarf our loudest intestinal rumblings and belches. Considering that most detoxification goes on at night, the noise of our sanitation department would surely keep us up if were able to give forth sounds comparable to the work it does. As it is, a faulty detoxification system is a common reason for poor sleep. We sometimes reach too quickly for a sedative for our nerves when it is our liver that needs help.

To understand the substantial portion of our daily expenditure of energy on all the chores of living that require making new molecules consider how it would go if the body were a municipality. The budget would look like this:

**Sanitation,** 80 percent (the various detoxication activities)
**Police,** 5 percent (the immune system)
**School system,** 10 percent (the central nervous system)
**Public works,** 6 percent (maintenance of organs)

Do not hold me to the exact figures except that the sanitation figure is, if anything, a conservative estimate. With a child who is devoting energy to making new molecules every day to grow, the budget would allocate relatively more for public works. No matter how you slice it, however, it is sobering to realize that most of the molecules we synthesize every day are made for the sake of getting rid of waste molecules.

## A Two-Step Operation

Before leaving the municipal analogy, let me make another general point about detoxification chemistry in preparation for a closer look at the details. It is a two-step operation. In my town the trash collection is done privately. For about a dollar a day, Harry Brasslett comes twice a week and takes away the trash, and on the second Wednesday of each month he comes for the recycling of bottles, cans, newspaper and cardboard. Like detoxification chemistry, the semiweekly trash and the monthly recycling are each two-phase operations. Phase one consists of making the trash easy to pick up. I place it in barrels or in plastic sacks and put it in a convenient location, protecting it from the raccoons until a few hours before Harry makes his rounds. In phase two Harry comes in his big white truck and takes it away. The success of the operation depends not only on the timely preparation of the trash but on a certain balance between the capacities of each phase. When we need to get rid of unwanted molecules from our bodies the first phase renders the molecules easy to pick up. "Sticky" is a better image. A system of enzymes called cytochrome P450 prepares leftover or toxic molecules and affects the molecules in a way that is very roughly like rubbing a balloon on your sweater. At this moment the molecules that have been made more sticky, or "activated," are more dangerous than they were to begin with. A sticky toxin is not something you want banging around in your chemistry. It is like flypaper in the barn. It is good to have the flies stick to the paper, but if the paper gets stuck in your hair it is worse than the flies were to begin with. The next step, then, is the timely appearance of the "Harry" molecules that carry the toxins away after safely containing them in a big white truck. Actually the process is called conjugation, and the more accurate image is sticking the sticky trash to individually tiny, somewhat sticky trucks. When each activated toxic or leftover molecule is stuck to a carrier molecule it becomes deactivated and more soluble in the water of your blood or bile so that it can leave your body via your kidneys or intestine.

The carrier molecules (the tiny trucks) owe their stickiness to properties familiar to anyone who has experience with sugar or garlic. In fact, two of the main carrier molecules are sticky because they are like sugar: one comes directly from sugar (glucuronide) and the other is an amino acid (glycine) that is sweet and sticky like sugar. Two other carrier molecules owe their stickiness to the same feature that makes garlic peels adhere to your fingers: sulfur. Sulfur is stinky and sticky. Sulfur atoms appear wherever stickiness is needed in chemistry, so they have an adhesive function in building strong tissues and sticking to waste molecules in your body's sanitation department.

The brimstone appearing in bright yellow deposits around the fumaroles of volcanoes is sulfur. It has unique properties. It is the only naturally occurring substance found lying about on the planet that can burn, but was not once alive. Other elements oxidize; that is, they combine with the oxygen in the air as in the tarnishing of silver or the rusting of iron. Still other elements, such as sodium and potassium, burn explosively so that if they are removed from the liquid in which they are stored in a chemistry lab and plunged directly into a flushing toilet, the ensuing blast will cause serious damage to the plumbing. But sodium and potassium are not just lying around on the planet. In nature they are tightly combined with other elements to form compounds (such as table salt: sodium and chlorine) which are quite harmless because of a mutual neutralization of the chemical ferocity of the two components.

The chemical ferocity of sulfur, however, is special. It has an avidity for other elements that is more in keeping with the kinds of avidity that hold together living flesh. It is a nonliving substance that has the character of living or once-living material: it burns. As such it has "the imponderable qualities of life, light, warmth"[75] and, indeed, it is indispensable to life and a critical component of the diet. If the body does not get enough of it, or if it misuses it, the detoxication systems and the synthesis and repair of tissue are impaired. Remember Queen Methionine. Her treasure consists of methyl groups as well as sulfur. Methionine is one of the principal ways that sulfur enters the body to become the most important adhesive that holds it together and helps it safely get rid of your toxins and leftovers.

## SOME HARMFUL TOXINS

**Aluminum:** Now let us follow the first sample toxin as it enters the body. Imagine that you have just enjoyed a delicious tomato sauce prepared in an aluminum pot. The acid sauce dissolved some of the pot's metallic aluminum, which entered your bloodstream with your meal. The body normally contains no aluminum, and aluminum does not resemble any atom that the body is used to handling. After all, metallic aluminum came into wide use only after the invention of a method for separating it from its ore in the nineteenth century. Aluminum, the most plentiful component of the rocks of the earth's crust, is abundant in our environment. Metallic aluminum, however, was virtually unknown to our species before this century. Aluminum has a particular affinity for phosphates that form an active part of our DNA. Instead of knocking electrons off the DNA like the shoe store X-ray machine might have done to mine, aluminum's affinity for the electrons of the phosphates of DNA simply makes it join up with DNA and get in the way. It does not leave. Once it is on board, it is essentially stuck there and does not leave the body. In fact, no matter what you do, your body will contain more aluminum at the time of your death than at any other time in your life.

Apart from its DNA-damaging effects, aluminum impairs a step in the citric acid cycle[76] where AKG is formed. Recall that AKG is one of the most useful workers in all of biochemistry, and you will understand the possible impact of having it weakened. Recall that other toxins, such as those described with Dr. Shaw's research in chapter 11, have the potential for interfering with AKG, and you will understand that many different toxins may have the same biochemical effects on people just as the same toxin may have many different clinical effects on different people. Exactly how much damage aluminum does to exactly what kinds of people remains controversial, but three things are certain: it is harmful,[77] there is no natural way to unload it and there is no proven treatment for the damage it causes at present.

Aluminum can be measured in hair, urine or blood and if an individual has too much on board he or she should look carefully for ways to avoid it, especially in cookware, some deodorants, some antacids and food additives. Unlike the monarch butterfly's helpful sequestration of its milkweed toxin, the aluminum toxin hides out just where it can do the most harm. The amino acid, glycine, helps mobilize aluminum in the body. An oral dose of 80 mg per kg of body weight of glycine, given in divided doses over a 24-hour period, is a noninvasive diagnostic test for drawing aluminum into the urine collected during that time. This test helps to determine how much aluminum is stored in the body. An experimental method for removing aluminum from the body involves the use of glycine combined with magnesium EDTA as a chelating agent.

**Lead:** Lead is one of the oldest, most ubiquitous and most insidious of toxins. Unlike aluminum it is greeted by the body as if it were familiar; it is treated as if it were calcium so its absorption is favored by calcium deficiency. Thus, symptoms of chronic lead poisoning, such as seizures, increase during the northern summer months when the increase of sunlight raises vitamin D levels to affect the mobilization of calcium and lead.

A form of lead, lead acetate, was the first artificial sweetener. No substance formed by a plant or animal is sweet unless it contains sugar. In the natural world you can depend on the rule that a food that is sweet is nourishing. The basis for the appreciation of sweet taste on the tongue is a certain distance between atoms of sugar molecules that is unique to sugars except for those molecules that have been formed artificially and have the identical interatomic spaces to fool the taste buds into a false perception of sweetness. Lead acetate happens to have such an atomic configuration, and it was used to sweeten wine during the Middle Ages until this form of food adulteration became a capital crime in Europe. Saccharine, extracted from coal tar, and other artificial sweeteners in current use represent less toxic ways of fooling the taste buds. However, I wonder if it is a good idea to repeatedly get the tongue to announce to the pancreas that sugar is on its way only to have the blood sugar-regulating mechanisms later surprised to find that the tongue's promise was empty. When I enter a supermarket and see the volume of diet soda on sale I realize that there is a lot of pancreatic trick or treating going on.

The worst trick comes from lead paint, which tastes sweet for the reasons just explained. A toddler finding chips of sweet-tasting material on a window sill or some other source of paint chips would naturally eat it, and so become poisoned, as the lead is widely distributed, like calcium, in the body's chemistry. Like aluminum it shows up in hair, which is the most convenient tissue used to screen for heavy metal toxicity. Precautions must be taken to collect hair correctly, using samplings close to the scalp and only hair that has not been treated. The body's biochemical efforts to get rid of lead typify all such efforts to unload unwanted exogenous toxins. First it is activated to make it sticky and then it is handed to reduced glutathione, which disappears along with the lead.

Treatment of lead poisoning begins with insuring adequate supplies of the substances the body uses naturally to carry out its removal, beginning with calcium to displace the lead and prevent the "hunger" for lead that is found when calcium supplies are short. Supplements of vitamin C, B vitamins and reduced glutathione may be sufficient to get rid of lead in mild cases of lead overload. Various chelating agents are used when the problem is severe or when there is a need to remove a number of heavy metals from the body. Chelation therapy, in which care must be taken to replace calcium, magnesium and other nutritional elements that are lost during treatment, is still denounced by medical authorities. I am not personally a practitioner of chelation therapy because it was outlawed by the Connecticut legislature for years and more recently my small office does not lend itself to such procedures. I believe that this and other methods to remove a toxic burden of heavy metals makes common sense and will eventually join the mainstream of medicine.

**Other toxins:** Let me turn to four other "toxins" that are used in tests to represent all unwanted molecules to determine how well the body can get rid of them:

- Caffeine (as found in coffee or over-the-counter stay-awake pills such as No-Doz)
- Acetaminophen (such as found in Tylenol and similar fever and pain medicines)
- Aspirin
- Sodium benzoate (a common food preservative)

By doing a test to follow these substances through the body, a good estimate of the efficiency of detoxification chemistry can be made. Making such an estimate provides a basis for judging the overall efficiency of a patient's body chemistry.

## TESTING THE DETOXIFICATION SYSTEM: A CASE STUDY

For example, here are the results of Mrs. Stockwell's detoxification tests for two of these four substances, taken both before and after her treatment with hydrocortisone.

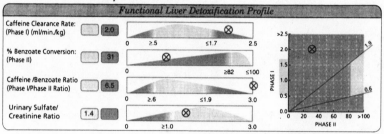

FIGURE 1

**Mrs. Stockwell's Detoxification Test: Before**

While these lab results, as they appear on the forms sent out by the laboratory,* resemble Seth's results shown in chapter 13, they portray entirely different information. In Figure 1, the top of the diagram shows how Mrs. Stockwell's detoxification systems handle caffeine. You can see that caffeine has a value of 2 ml/min/kg, which is above the normal range of .5 to 1.7. Figure 2 shows her caffeine clearance rate after six weeks of treatment for her adrenal insufficiency. It has fallen to a normal value of 1.7. Her benzoate clearance went from a markedly low value of 31 percent to a squarely normal value of 87 percent. The net effect of the two changes is shown in the third row of the graphics as well as in the graph on the right side of each test result, indicating a normalization of the relationship between the two results.

Here is what was done to get these results. For each test Mrs.

---

* Great Smokies Diagnostic Laboratory, 18 A Regent Park Boulevard, Asheville, North Carolina 28806

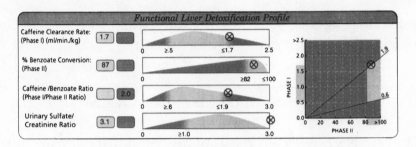

FIGURE 2

Mrs. Stockwell's Detoxification Test: After

Stockwell was given a kit to use at home with a dose of caffeine (one No-Doz pill) and a dose of sodium benzoate, a safe chemical used in many foods. After avoiding all foods containing either substance as well as an overnight fast, she took both test materials with a glass of water and then collected her urine for the following six hours. Her urine was subsequently analyzed at the laboratory to show what had become of the two substances. The detoxification of caffeine depends heavily on the detoxification step in which toxins are made sticky or activated by the enzyme system, cytochrome P450. There are many members of the P450 team, each specializing in different kinds of toxins, and caffeine gives a reasonable test of one of the main members of the team. Sodium benzoate tests phase II of the detoxication process in which the carrier, in this case the amino acid glycine, is conjugated with the toxin (sodium benzoate) to remove it safely from the body. As you will see presently, the test for evaluating detoxification chemistry has been improved since Mrs. Stockwell took the tests diagrammed in Figures 1 and 2. The laboratory now provides a more comprehensive look at other parts of phase II of the detoxification process, parts that involve other sugar-sticky carriers as well as two sulfur-sticky ones. In Mrs. Stockwell's case the test as performed was sufficient to show how much better her detoxification chemistry was working at the same time that she was feeling better. The evidence of the usefulness of these tests and others I will mention is published widely in the scientific literature. The appropriate references for each of the many tests are available from Great Smokies Laboratory, Asheville, NC. I show Mrs. Stockwell's results only as an illustrative example. Considering that nothing about Mrs. Stockwell's diet or other treatments changed except in the ways I described, it is particularly interesting that the second test changed as it did. The amount of sulfur in its form of sulfate that came out in her urine is a fair reflection of the sufficiency of this important component of her detoxification chemistry. The result of her "before" test was toward the lower end of normal. After treatment she showed a robust and healthy rise in sulfate excretion to the upper limits of what is expected. Somewhat high levels of excretion are okay. Low levels, reflecting inadequate amounts of sulfur-containing detoxification chemicals, are undesirable.

The test has now been improved to include two other substances (aspirin and acetaminophen or Tylenol®) whose detoxification pathways involve all of the carriers, including two sulfur-sticky ones: reduced glutathione and plain sulfate and another sugar-sticky carrier called glucuronic acid. See Figure 3 on the next page. The three test substances are shown at the top of the diagram. Below caffeine is its clearance result and below acetaminophen and salicylic acid (aspirin) are figures showing how much of each was recovered unchanged from the patient's urine.

## THE VALUE OF STOOL TESTS

The intestine, which is both the passageway and the source of important toxins, also plays an important role in detoxification. Therefore, stool tests are a top priority in assessing health and detecting the cause of health problems. A wealth of information can be extracted from stool if it is submitted to careful biochemical, microscopic and microbiological examination. Here are the basics:

**1. Digestion.** It is common sense that good digestion of food is a prerequisite to good health. People may have relatively comfortable digestion even when it is not working well at the functional level. In this sense digestion refers quite specifically to the process I described in chapter 7. Examination of a stool sample under the microscope reveals whether meat and/or vegetable fibers have survived their pas-

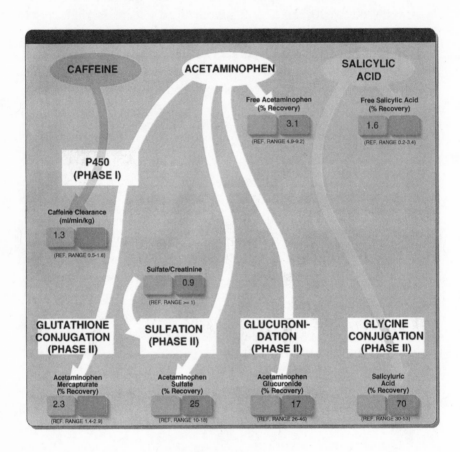

FIGURE 3

### Detoxification Markers

sage through the intestine in undue numbers. Most of us are familiar with the capacity of corn kernels to make it through in recognizable form. They owe this capability to their surrounding coat of indigestible cellulose fiber which shield the nourishing inner material from the digestive process unless the kernel is initially well broken up by chewing. Most of the other grains we eat would do the same thing but we don't eat many other grains "on the cob."

A biochemical assessment of the stool also reveals how well fat has been digested. Very little fat of any kind (cholesterol, triglycerides, free fatty acids) should make it through the gut. Fat may vary in the stool from time to time, so the best test to really quantify fat in the stool requires a 72-hour collection. Not a popular test, but fat analysis in a random specimen is an adequate first step.

**2. The nutrition of the gut.** The cells that line the surface of the intestinal tract require nourishment as do all of the cells of the body. They are different from all the other cells of the body, however, in that they live where food is passing by. Do they need to wait for that food to pass into the circulation and then to be delivered to them, through the back door so to speak, just as any normal cell would be nourished from the blood's distribution? Or could the cells of the digestive tract grab a bite from the passing food stream?

The digestive tract's total surface area is about the size of a tennis court. It's job is absorbing all of the nutrients and excluding toxins while being subject to the wear and tear of passing food and the toxic effects of germs that inhabit or easily invade the warm, moist, nutrient-dense environment of the gut. The care and feeding of the short-lived cells of the intestine's lining is of particular importance in the overall task of the care and feeding of the permanent, essential cells described in chapter 1. Nature has provided for the intestinal cells to be able to "eat" food that passes by without waiting for some nutrients to be delivered back to them via the bloodstream after passing through the liver. The cells of the large intestine are provided with small, nourishing molecules that are produced as the germs of the digestive tract process fiber. Germs break down the fiber into very small molecules with only two, three or four carbon atoms called acetate, propionate and butyrate respectively. Acetate is familiar to you in the taste of vinegar, and butyrate in the taste of butter. Propionate is found in milk and as a preservative in bread and is also used in making perfumes. None of these foods, however, is the source of the acetate, propionate and butyrate used by the cells that line the intestine. These cells depend on healthy, normal bacteria to process the fiber in the diet into these nutrients. In the upper digestive tract, where there are very few germs, the cells use the amino acid glutamine as part of their nourishment.

**3. pH.** I referred previously to the acidifying effect of carbon dioxide, whether it be from an actual fire or the sort made by living metabolism. I also referred to ammonia as an amino acid (and protein) breakdown product that requires costly metabolic measures to insure its conversion in our body to the safe by-product urea. When germs, such as the ones that live in the intestine, metabolize amino acids they just make ammonia and are done with it. The consequence of the combined activities of germs making acid in the "smoke" from their metabolic fire and ammonia from the breakdown of amino acid is a compromise between the alkalinity of ammonia and the acidity of the metabolism. As a result, stool is normally quite close to the neutral pH of 7 or a little below, say down to 6 on the scale that measures the concentration of acid. Low numbers indicate more acid, and high numbers indicate alkalinity. The pH of stomach acid is about 1, which is 100,000,000 times more acid than 7 since it is based on a log scale, where each point represents a 10-fold increase or decrease. The acidity of the stool has nothing to do with the acidity of the blood and tissues. It is entirely the product of bacterial fermentation and the balance between germs with different appetites and by-products. An acid stool indicates the presence of too much food entering the lower intestine for the germs to digest and strongly suggests that the food passed undigested into the stool from the upper part of the digestive tract. An alkaline stool indicates the presence of unfriendly germs with a strong ammonia-producing capability.

**4. Microbiology.** Of the few hundred different kinds of germs that inhabit the digestive tract, only a few can be easily identified on routine cultures. About half (the germs that thrive where there is no oxygen) do not show up on cultures unless special procedures are taken. Among the other half (the so-called aerobic germs) a few of the predominant friendly bacteria should be present in stool cultures to indicate a healthy balance. These are *lactobacillus* (also known as acidophilus), *bifidobacter, E. coli, bacillus* species, *gamma strep* and a few others. Among the other germs that appear in a stool culture are some whose presence automatically indicates an infection, but for the most part the overgrowth of various unwanted germs is indicated not by their presence, but by the excessive numbers of certain kinds that usually represent a small, smelly minority. As a general rule, the odor of stools is an indication of its germs' capacity to cause mischief. The stronger the odor of stools and intestinal gas, the greater the indication of unwanted fermentation in the gut.

In Africa I was involved in projects to encourage the earlier feeding of solid foods to children who were about to be weaned from an exclusive breast milk diet at around age two. Since weaning is a time of major stress when children often lose weight and are susceptible to serious illness, the gradual introduction of solid food a few months ahead of time was intended to give the child nutritional support. In Africa nursing babies and young children spend a good deal of time on their mothers' backs supported by a broad cloth. Thus, the close physical connection between mother and child affords reliable signals when a baby is about to have a bowel movement. This provides the opportunity for the mother to remove the baby from her back, hold it in the appropriate position to have a bowel movement, clean the baby off, and then return it to its accustomed spot. Diapers, diaper rash and all the other complications engendered by a baby sitting in its own stool are unknown in the setting where I worked. The well-meaning and healthy steps that we recommended to the women of the village caused a disturbance in the timing and the odor of their babies' stools. The result was ill-timed, stinky stools that came without warning and soiled baby, mother and cloth. Breast-fed babies' stools have an inoffensive odor characteristic of the *lactobacillus* and other friendliest of germs that inhabit them. As soon as some other kind of food is introduced, such as cow's milk, formula or solids, the stool takes on the odor of an adult's, which is unwelcome in any setting.

The two lessons drawn from this are: 1) One cannot always anticipate all the consequences of well-meaning efforts to change long-standing practices and habits, and 2) the nose is a pretty good guide to intestinal function. Thus, if the odor of your stools is particularly offensive you do not need a stool test to alert you that something is wrong with the balance of odor-causing germs that inhabit your intestine.

**5. Mycology and parasitology.** Fungi are larger, more complex and completely different kinds of germs than bacteria. The fungi that normally constitute a very small percentage of the gut flora are yeasts. Sometimes other kinds of fungi can be found in stools. The term parasite is used by doctors to denote a great variety of creatures that vary in size and complexity from single-celled organisms that are close to being fungi all the way up to worms that may be several inches or more in length. The smaller the germ the more virulent it is likely to be (i.e., a virus as compared to a worm). As is true with any germ, the trouble starts when the immune system starts to fight back. Symptoms develop not from the germ, so to speak, but from the fight. Some parasites awaken very little response on the part of the immune system, which may only take on an attitude of chronic irritation in the presence of an unwanted passenger. The spectrum of symptoms evoked by parasites can vary, therefore, from intense diarrhea (dysentery) such as I frequently encountered in my patients in Africa to a complete lack of symptoms in the digestive tract but with inflammation elsewhere in the body.

In the last 20 years I have changed my ideas more about parasites than just about any other topic that comes up in my medical practice. When I left the tropics in the late 1960s and returned to North America I thought that my knowledge of parasitology would get little further use. Part of that knowledge was that there are several "minor" parasites that are of relatively little consequence to the health of their human hosts, who tolerate the presence of the microbe without much objection and therefore with few symptoms unless the immune system is impaired. I carried an attitude engendered by the tropical environment where, indeed, the object was to take care of the big-league parasites that cause serious illness. About the time I returned from Africa, *giardiasis* became much more prevalent in North America. It could not be considered a minor parasite as it often causes serious illness. Sometimes it is quite silent and hard to find so that its detection, like the detection of other single-celled parasites, requires a very high degree of laboratory expertise and experience.

The same expertise is needed to find other parasites that I was taught to ignore until I started learning to pay more attention to them from colleagues such as Dr. Warren Levin in New York City, who had been influenced by two New York parasitologists, Dr. Louis Parrish and Dr. Herman Bueno, who later worked with my friend and former partner Dr. Leo Galland. Dr. Galland has become a leading expert in the relationship between parasitic problems and chronic disease. His paper, *Intestinal Dysbiosis and the Cause of Disease,*[78] coauthored by Dr. Stephen Barrie, founder of Great Smokies Laboratory, includes a completely referenced survey of the problem. Looking for *giardia,* I came up with reports of what I had previously believed to be innocent parasites on the lab reports I received along with a microscopic picture of the patient's stool showing the parasite.

*Blastocystis hominis* is the most common of such parasites and now, after more than 10 years of seeing and treating hundreds of patients with this parasite, I am convinced that it should be eradicated when found. When stool is examined for parasites, most of the yeasts that are seen there are dead. Yeast cultures, therefore, frequently fail to reveal the presence of fungi even when the gut is heavily colonized. A negative stool culture is, therefore, not an indication of the absence of yeast. The tests being developed by Dr. Shaw, mentioned earlier, may help solve the problem of detecting significant numbers of yeast. However, the meaning of "significant" varies from individual to individual, so that the only decisive way to diagnose a yeast problem is by giving a trial of treatment with antifungal medication.

**6. Gut immunity.** The intestine is by far the largest and most complex frontier on which the body encounters its environment. The internal surface of the lungs is of similar size but is incomparably cleaner. Most of the resources of the immune system are concentrated on the gut where most of the antibodies made every day are used to label and inactivate foreign substances as they are encountered. Label and inactivate: these are the two jobs of antibodies which are globular-shaped protein molecules (hence globulins) that are used as the immune system perceives its environment.

As I explained in chapter 1, recognition is something we do with our central nervous system as well as our immune system.

When we perceive something with the eyes, ears, skin, tongue or nose it is a one-step operation. As we behold something, we know it. The immune system's perception of things is more of a two-step operation. First a sticky label is placed on the scrutinized object to simultaneously inactivate it and mark it. Then a label-reader cell is able to identify it and spread the word to the rest of the immune system. The most abundant immune globulins that are made every day are produced in the intestine in a collaborative effort of the cells that make antibodies (lymphocytes), aided by cells that line the intestinal wall. The name of this antibody is secretory IgA, which can be measured in saliva, milk and other secretions of the body, but now is being measured by Great Smokies Laboratory as part of its comprehensive stool examination. Secretory IgA levels are elevated in the presence of infection or overgrowth of unwelcome germs and are depressed if the infection or overgrowth is excessive. Some individuals are born with an incapacity to produce secretory IgA and they subsequently have more problems with infection and allergy.

When I first evaluated Dr. Franco's detoxification systems I found enough yeast in her stool culture to raise the question of an overgrowth of Candida affecting her immune and endocrine systems. The endocrine effects of Candida are dramatic, and infertility, in my experience, is a common consequence. At the same time I measured her 24-hour urine amino acids. Influenced by Dr. Rosenberg to be aware of the potential importance of amino acid metabolism in severe disorders, I was impressed by two papers that appeared in the pediatric literature in the early 1970s reporting a marked difference in the serum amino acid patterns in breast-fed versus formula-fed babies. If amino acid analysis could be used to measure such "normal" differences based on diets that were intended to be comparable, I wondered whether amino acid analysis could be used to spot other differences in the metabolism of individuals whose biochemical quirks did not reach the level of disease but might indicate they would benefit from nutritional intervention.

In the mid-1970s I had heard stories from a number of patients who reported benefits to their health from taking vitamins. Some of the stories were very striking, such as the remission of long-standing severe recurring migraine after taking supplements of vitamin B6 and magnesium. I knew quite well from my medical training that vitamins and magnesium were not the treatment for migraine but yet this combination worked for this individual. I was terrified to think that I would have to go back and learn all the biochemistry that I had mostly forgotten after my board exams and jumped at the chance to take courses called "Basic Science for Clinicians" under the leadership of Dr. Edward Rubenstein at Stanford University Medical School.

There were five Nobel laureates on the faculty, including Linus Pauling. Meeting Dr. Pauling and attending his lectures changed my life, allowing me to realize that the basic principles of biochemistry were accessible. He gave me the courage to move ahead and accumulate the details as I went along. The details of amino acid chemistry remained relatively overwhelming until I met Jon Pangborn, Ph.D. Dr. Pangborn had plunged into the biochemistry literature motivated to understand the biochemical quirks that had been revealed when his autistic son had come up with abnormalities that did not fit any known pattern but were too out of line to be considered normal variations. In the 25 years that have elapsed since then, Dr. Pangborn has become a unique resource for the understanding of published biochemistry literature as it applies to the search for individual patterns that may not constitute diseases but which give leverage in balancing individual chemistry. His work exemplifies a phenomenon that is implicit in the tone and content of this book and which I will digress to describe briefly here.

There is only one immunology and only one biochemistry. There are, however, two camps in medicine. Disease-oriented medicine and individual-oriented medicine* do not differ on the current facts of biochemistry and immunology. The difference is entirely one of orientation. Disease-oriented medicine is directed to finding the generalized formulas for treating groups of people who resemble one another in certain symptomatic respects. Such an approach is

---

* Dr. Galland's "patient-centered diagnosis" or Dr. Jeffrey Bland's "functional medicine" are other terms for this approach.

indispensable to thoughtful medical practice. Individual-oriented medicine's approach is to find everything possible that can be done to optimize the health of a given unique individual. Such an approach is also indispensable to thoughtful medical practice and it requires a disquieting degree of judgment to know when individual differences are significant enough to treat. As I said earlier, if you do enough tests you can find something wrong with just about anyone. This phrase goes to the core of the medical dichotomy. In one camp is the attitude that whatever is found wrong must rise above individuality to join a pattern linked to a group of people who all have "the same thing." In the other camp is the attitude that an effort should be made to harmonize a patient's chemistry when it is clearly abnormal even though the abnormality does not constitute a disease. Amino acid chemistry gives such good insight into a broad range of activities involving minerals, vitamins and amino acids that it provides the most sensitive gauge of biochemical harmony available to physicians interested in individuality. It will become more commonly used over the next few years as Dr. Pangborn's approach and skills become more widely used by others.

When I evaluated Dr. Franco's amino acids in chapter 2 there was an overall pattern of numerous very high or very low values. It did not look like a normal variation nor a disease. Among several findings was an especially low level of all of the sulfur-containing amino acids that participate in detoxification: the children, so to speak, of methionine. From the cyberhealth perspective it would be reasonable but speculative to take nontoxic steps to improve this part of her chemistry through, for example, supplements that would augment her supply of reduced glutathione. That is what was done. From a mainstream perspective an allegiance to the scientific approach would suggest that the treatment of her yeast problem and her detoxification should take place separately so that "we will know what is doing what."

From the cyberhealth perspective we can see a logical connection between both abnormalities (and some others as well) and the status of her reproductive chemistry. An allegiance to the need to do everything possible (and safe) and to cover all the bases led to the combined treatments that were associated with her pregnancy. As is often the case in this approach, we will never know exactly what, if anything, worked. When I first became interested in this approach to medicine I did not think it would work very often but it was worth a try for the sake of covering all the bases for my patient. I was surprised to find that it usually works and that people actually do get better.

## THE ROLE OF OXIDATIVE STRESS

Most of the tests I have referred to so far measure a kind of problem that can be localized to a particular place in the body or its digestive, immune and biochemical processes. What about testing for damage by oxidative stress, which could show up anywhere from the fatty acids in sunburned skin on the tip of the nose to the nucleic acids in the DNA of cells that are destined for conceiving a child? Oxidative damage, the loss of electrons from molecules who lose a tug-of-war with oxygen or other electron-hungry thieves, takes place everywhere, but its effects might be felt in different ways depending on the life span and location of, say, the skin cells or the reproductive system. As I described previously, the fatty acids of the cell membranes are some of the most susceptible to the theft of their electrons. Packed together like millions of caterpillars standing on their tails, the oxidation of one of them yields a domino effect among its neighbors. The magnification of damage caused by the domino effect makes fatty acids (also known under the collective term lipids) good objects of analysis to see how much oxidative stress the body has endured without being able to defend itself with the team of antioxidants, including vitamin C, the flavonoids, beta-carotene, vitamin E and reduced glutathione. Just as I pointed out that this partnership of chemicals works as a team, it is appropriate to neither give one team member alone as a treatment nor to measure one member as a way of assessing the efficiency of the whole team. Consequently we either need to measure all of these substances, which can be done in a blood specimen, or we can measure the effect of the team's failure. Blood tests for rancid fatty acids (or lipid peroxides) are the best direct measure of oxidative damage. Another good test involves adding a step to the detoxification test I described earlier in which caffeine, acetaminophen and aspirin are run through the system to see how well they are detoxified. If blood as well as urine is used for analysis, the by-products of the body's handling of aspirin can be used to assess the degree of oxidative stress inside cells.

The development of the aspirin test for oxidative stress as well as future tests[79] to evaluate other key indicators of cellular health and oxidative stress (e.g., nitric oxide) is largely the work of Jeffrey Bland, Ph.D. Between the lines of this book you can find the birth record of a new paradigm of medicine that is coming into being. Dr. Bland has been the principal midwife of this delivery. He has been and continues to be the preeminent educator of physicians whose appetite for biochemistry and immunology has been whetted by their need to study their patients as individuals. Thousands of patients have benefited directly from the knowledge that Dr. Bland has brought to their physicians with a flawless sense for applying a rigorous, detailed understanding of biochemistry to a systems approach to medicine and a superlative knack for explaining things.

I went to medical school after graduating from college with a history degree, and my step-father, Henry Bragdon, and my uncle, Thomas C. Mendenhall, both had long careers as historians. As I try to imagine how our present medical position will be seen when today becomes history I cannot quite see how medicine aimed at treating people as individuals will break out of the bondage of the current system in which the medical specialties, insurance companies, the pharmaceutical industry and research funds are so entirely focused on diseases. Whatever happens, however, I am sure that Jeffrey Bland will stand out as a key teacher of the evolving theory and practice of the new paradigm. Dr. Bland and I have spent many hours trying to combine our different approaches to teaching so that the mix of stories and hard data may be mutually beneficial in getting the message across. If I have awakened your interest in the subject at hand, you will want to read Dr. Bland's new book, *The 20-Day Rejuvenation Diet Program.*

There is no one specific way for everyone to detoxify his or her body, whether by fasting, drinking lots of vegetable juices, sweating or taking vitamins. The method for detoxification may depend entirely on some particular factor that is quite peculiar to the individual and will depend on an assessment of food sensitivities, whether or not the body has an excess burden of particular toxins from exogenous poisons or endogenous microbes, or whether or not the digestive tract is functioning properly. There are, however, a few simple steps that apply to many people.

The first is to avoid allergenic foods. These foods may be determined by blood tests as I described earlier or by trying an experimental two-week trial of what Dr. William Crook calls the Caveman Diet[81] in which most allergenic foods are avoided such as eggs, grains, dairy and citrus to see if it makes a difference in symptoms. The second is the use of the hypoallergenic, nutrient-dense food product, UltraClear, designed by Dr. Bland. There are several forms of UltraClear, and you will need some guidance in choosing the correct one. The intent of the UltraClear products is to support the chemistry of both phases of detoxification as well as to help heal the bowel by providing nutrients, fiber and normal flora to the gut. Its value in doing the things it is supposed to do has been documented experimentally[82] and I have seen dramatic changes in patients' symptoms as well as their laboratory tests with its use. It shares with fasting the advantage of removing the load of allergens from the gut, but it has the advantage of not depriving the body of essential nutrients when the body is trying to accomplish a nutritionally demanding task.

CHAPTER 16

# Rhythmic Harmony and Breathing

TAKE A DEEP BREATH and prepare for a change of pace and viewpoint. So far, we have looked at biochemistry as if it were frozen in time. It is not. In the time you took to take and release a deep breath you broke the rhythm of your breathing and in the same moment you changed your chemistry a little as well. The acidity of your blood fell as you exhaled the carbon dioxide smoke from your metabolic fire, and your chemistry made transient subtle shifts as it awaited the high tide of your next breath. Our bodies and our lives revolve around rhythms that are harmonious and predictable. When these rhythms are fully integrated, we achieve a healthy harmony. We become less fit when the rhythms are not synchronized.

Let us start with an image. Picture a swing. Picture a brilliant sunny day. Now put a child on the swing. You stand behind and provide the push. Whether you are gently pushing a small child or a big child aiming for treetops, there is a kind of perfect push that feels "right." The swing rises to meet your hands, your hands yield to the swing's motion as the swing and hands meet and the push of the hands returns the swing to its next arc. The pusher's hands and the child's body each know when the push is just right and when it's a little off. When the push is just right the pusher can rest until the child has made four, five or six excursions into the sky. Then the pusher can renew the momentum with another perfectly timed push. A perfect push of the 35-foot swing on my big oak tree will last for four oscillations for Andrew, five for Michael and Liana and six for Aidan, who is the smallest. The number of oscillations may vary with the size of the child, but, for perfect pushes, it is always exactly five, six, or seven and not, say five-and-a-half, which would find the child in the wrong place in time and space for any sort of reasonable push. When the timing of the pushes is just right, the integration of the swing and the pushes is harmonious and efficient. When the timing is off, both the pusher and the child lose a sense of efficiency and satisfaction. The numerical relationship and the timing of harmony permit no compromise. There would never be a situation in which efficiency would be gained by trying to stop the child in mid-air for a push at say 5.7 or 6.1 oscillations. The whole number (that is 5 and not 5.7, or 6 and not 6.1) relationships are unforgiving. When a rhythmically integrated system loses harmony, the result is disorder and inefficiency.

Take another deep breath. Depending on your respiratory rate and the speed of your reading it is the 60th, 78th, 100th or some "in-between" breath you have taken since I asked you to take a deep breath at the beginning of this chapter. Doctors call a respiratory rate of 18 breaths per minute normal because healthy adults' breathing does not vary much from individual to individual. There is, however, no ideal number of breaths to take per minute, and your own breathing will vary with your activity. The web of harmony in your body that I would like you to understand does not have to do with the relationship between your respiration or other rhythmic bodily activities and the clock. It has to do with the interrelationships of different rhythmic activities and the effect of breathing on those relationships.

Some rhythmic activities of your body are: nerve impulses, ciliary action, brain waves, heartbeat, respiration and peristalsis. Every day your body goes through a cycle (the circadian rhythm) in which waking and sleeping are the outward expressions of an entire sequence of biochemical rhythms. Longer rhythms are expressed on a monthly (menstrual) and seasonal (annual) basis, and there are even slower cycles that have to do with the stages of one's development as a person. Our biological rhythms are hierarchically structured so that "every rapid and more specialized rhythm is at the same time part of a slower and more embracing process."[83]

Later we will look at breathing as the key to healthy rhythms. In the meantime, let us look at a specific example that will lead to an understanding of how rhythm can be more or less toxic or healthy. In the article from which the above quote was taken, the author, Dr. G. Hildebrandt reports the following experiment. Volunteers did a standardized exercise in which they climbed the same three steps six times in one minute. Each subject's heart and respiratory rates were taken at rest and at 30-second intervals during the first five minutes of recovery after the exercise. Subjects were scored by their rate of recovery—how quickly they return to their resting pulse and respiratory rates. Such scores are taken as a measure of fitness. Each subject's average respiratory rate and average heart rate were calculated over the five-minute recovery time. For example, one subject might have had an average respiratory rate of 25 and a heart rate of 100. Another subject might also have had a respiratory rate of 25 but a heart rate of 87. If you think of the heart rate as if it were the pusher of the swing and the breathing rate as the child on the swing, then the first subject's relationship is analogous to Andrew on the swing: one push for every four swings or one breath every four heart beats (25 breaths for every 100 heart beats, 100 divided by 25 equals 4). The harmony of the timing makes a difference in the same way that the harmony of pushing a swing makes a difference.

Let us look at the second subject. His breathing rate was 25 breaths and his heart rate was 87 on average. The relationship between those two rates is 25 to 87: 87 divided by 25 equals 3.48. Of the 140 subjects tested by Dr. Hildebrandt, 24 had relationships between their pulse and respiration rates that averaged out to whole numbers and the others had relationships that fell in between. Eleven subjects had a pulse/respiration ratio of 4; five subjects had a ratio of 5 and nine subjects had a ratio of 6. Other subjects had ratios such as 3.48, 4.3, 4.8 or 5.7 and so on. Remember that the test was one that measures physical fitness. Therefore we can compare the fitness of the subjects with different pulse/respiration ratios. The results of the experiment show a consistent and marked superiority of fitness for the subjects with whole-number ratios (especially 4 and 5) over those whose ratios fell in between. The conclusion is that a state of harmony between two different rhythms in the body is associated with a higher degree of fitness.

The point of this conclusion is that rhythmic disharmony can act like a toxin in the body. We can use this information to promote harmony in our rhythms when we realize that our respiratory rate is partly under our control. Or, to put it another way, if we let ourselves relinquish control of our breathing so that it joins the natural rhythms of the body, we will enjoy a higher level of health. Knowing about detoxification is not beneficial without understanding that good breathing is one of the main pivots on which health turns. Details about much of the information in this book are available from sources that disseminate knowledge about food, supplements or laboratory tests to doctors and to the public. Good breathing is more elusive. Before I present it to you, I would like to give you a broader context in which to think about rhythms.

When it comes to rhythms we are all the same. Throughout the book I have emphasized that individuality governs and complicates all our efforts to find a healthy balance in our biochemistry. The right dose of this or that medication, supplement or food for one person is not the right dose for another person. One person's meat is another person's poison. When it comes to rhythms, however, we all dance to the beat of the cycles of night and day which embrace the rhythms of sleeping, waking, eating and excreting.

Bowel movements are also rhythmic, not only in the peristaltic sense, but in the circadian sense. They should be at least daily just as the cycle of sleeping and waking should adhere to the cycle of night and day. When it comes to night and day, we are all the same. We may require different lengths of sleep, but we are all bound by the rhythm of the same cycle, which rocks in the cradle of our planet's rotation.

Unlike other creatures we can choose to depart from the environmental schedule, but not without paying a certain price. Just as we can hold the breath or control its rate for a while, we can decide to stay up all night. I did so many times as an intern and resident and paid the price when I nodded off as the lights were dimmed for slides at a conference the following day. My body was obedient to the rule: sleep in darkness and waken in daylight.

Many people get out of sorts when doing regular night work even though they sleep in a dark room during the day. Body chemistry retains its link to the planet's activities and does not adjust well to the simulation of light at night or darkness in the day. Shifting schedules are particularly difficult especially if the shift changes occur at frequent intervals so that the individual's body has insufficient time for even a partial adaptation.

The nuclear power plant accident at Three Mile Island was at four o'clock in the morning, the time of day when night workers are least alert. In the control room, where confusion turned an error into a disaster, the workers on duty had just started a new rotation of their shifting work schedule. The utility's policy was to rotate shifts in the "wrong direction," leaving workers particularly susceptible to fatigue and mental confusion. The difference between "right" and "wrong" direction of work shifts is the same as for travelers, who can adjust more quickly to jet lag when they fly across five time zones from New York to Hawaii than they can when they travel eastward over five time zones to England. A worker who is used to, or getting used to, working a 7 a.m. to 3 p.m. shift will have more difficulty adjusting to the earlier 11 p.m. to 7 a.m. shift than to the later 3 p.m. to 11 p.m. shift. The length of time that it takes to adjust in either case is greatly influenced by the timing of meals, the carbohydrate versus protein composition of meals, light exposure, social activity, and especially the timing intake of caffeine.[84] The timing of such factors can be used to greatly reduce the toxicity of jet lag and rotating shift work. The effective use of such timing to help in adjusting to the new beat is, in some instances, counterintuitive and requires study. For example, avoiding caffeine and eating a high protein breakfast (fish, cheese, eggs, meat) and a high carbohydrate dinner (pasta, bread, potatoes) favors adaptation to a new time zone. Nevertheless, most New Yorkers arriving in Paris after a night on the plane consume a continental breakfast of bread and jam and coffee and eat their protein in the evening. The military requirement to transport troops across great distances and arrive braced for battle has led to a substantial body of research that can benefit all travelers. It is summarized in a very useful volume[85] sold in most airport book shops.

The problems of travelers and shift workers illustrate the way that the most insistent of environmental rhythms, the day/night cycle, is the "push" and we are the children on a swing. Harmony exists when the timing of our swing is appropriate to the inflexible push of the physical world in which we live. Travelers as well as infants who are adjusting to the cycles of light and dark in their new environment outside the womb have obvious problems with their circadian rhythms. People with sleep disturbances may get help by taking a cue from the remedies for jet lag: light during the day, dark at night, protein in the morning, carbohydrate in the evening and abstinence from caffeine except perhaps at "teatime" in the afternoon, when it has a neutral influence, pushing the metabolic clock neither forward nor backward. These measures will help us stay tuned to the environment's swing.

Now let us return to the other rhythm: breathing. If you have trained your breath for singing or playing a wind instrument or if you have practiced yoga, then you know how to breathe with your diaphragm. Babies do so naturally. As people age they tend to change their breathing habits. The muscles of the upper chest lift the rib cage to expand the lungs and the diaphragm becomes less involved in the effort. The muscles of the upper chest normally function to provide the extra reserve of respiratory effort needed for exercise and they often become engaged when we are under stress. If, especially under stress, we can learn to let our diaphragm do our breathing, then the body works better. For example, if I am in an awkward position at the top of a ladder trying to drive a nail, I may find myself holding my breath as I line things up and then hit my thumb with the hammer. If I say to myself, "Relax, take the tension out of your chest and let your diaphragm do your breathing," the nail will probably go in with far less chance of damage to the thumb, the nail or the wood. Many people go about their waking activities as if they are up a ladder driving nails. Only when they sleep do they release their control over the rhythm of breathing so that it becomes regular and so that it can regain its natural integration with the rhythm of the heart.

The diaphragm muscle is a thin sheet draped over the top of the liver at the upper part of the abdomen. It makes a compete seal on all of its edges where it connects to the inside of the abdominal and chest cavity and provides a closed space for the lungs. When the diaphragm muscle contracts it flattens, its dome descends and the lungs expand to take up the space left by the diaphragm's travel. The downward movement of the center of the diaphragm acts as a plunger on the liver, stomach and intestines so that a deep diaphragmatic breath pushes the stomach out. Look in any magazine advertisement that features pictures of people that everyone supposedly wants to look like. Does any model have a stomach that sticks out? No. Everyone sticks the chest out and holds in the stomach.

Chronic stress, modern ideals of bodily attractiveness and ignorance about how to breathe properly all contribute to people breathing in a way that borders on holding the breath. It affects the metabolism in that it prevents the normal escape of carbon dioxide via the breath. That effect is subtle compared to the effect that chest breathing has on the integration of respiratory rhythms with the heart. The best way to address the problem is not with a deliberate effort to time the breath, but with an effort to make a habit of breathing with the diaphragm. The diaphragm is connected to centers in the brain that know about the heart rate. The chest muscles are not connected in this way. With correct breathing, the diaphragm will tend to establish a natural integration with the heart rate that is characteristic of the fit subjects in Dr. Hildebrandt's experiments. If the diaphragm takes over the breathing process, then the efficiency of all bodily activities will increase. Breathing diaphragmatically when performing any stressful activity, whether it is sitting for hours in front of a computer or running a mile, will enhance your performance.

I first learned about breathing when I was in India and Nepal and got my first lessons in Ayurvedic medicine. The importance of diaphragmatic breathing finally sunk in, however, when I made a brief effort at playing the recorder. My teacher asked me to lie on my back on the floor and emit a long, slow note with my voice. As I learned to keep my chest out of the effort and allow my diaphragm to descend to take in my breath, my note lasted longer and longer. Soon after I discovered that such lessons were not just for rank beginners like myself. A well-known clarinetist who has his own orchestra explained that he continued to take lessons in breathing and had done so under the guidance of a respiratory physiologist known as "Dr. Breath." In his book[86] on the subject, Dr. Breath reports the extraordinary improvement in the performance of athletes such as the U.S. track team for the 1968 Olympic Games, whom he coached in diaphragmatic breathing techniques. The improved performance is, I am sure, due not only to better oxygenation but to the harmony achieved when the diaphragm tunes itself to heart rate and the other cadences of the body.

# CHAPTER 17

# Some Final Thoughts

MY MENTOR, Dr. Shannon Brunjes, introduced me to one of the most influential essays I have ever read, written by Dr. F. G. Crookshank. It appears as an appendix in Ogden and Richards's classic treatise on language, *The Meaning of Meaning*.[87] When I first read it I was still a regular attendee at such medical school teaching conferences as Grand Rounds and Clinico-Pathological Conferences (CPC) which are well-known to all who are familiar with medical education. The phrase, "disease entity," is uttered at these conferences with a regularity that becomes distressing to anyone who has read Dr. Crookshank's essay "The Importance of a Theory of Signs and a Critique of Language in the Study of Medicine." A physician who read the essay at the time of its publication might be lost in the technology and pharmacology of today's medicine and be amazed and pleased with the many changes that allow physicians to save and prolong lives. The same physician would also probably be struck by our presently emerging capacity to study and make use of our knowledge of the individual differences in patients. I think that he or she would be surprised, however, that the problems discussed in Dr. Crookshank's essay have only gotten worse. Those problems have to do with the way we speak about illness (e.g., "disease entity"), the way we approach health problems and, according to Dr. Crookshank, a certain confusion about words, thoughts and things (or names, notions and happenings).

For example, *diabetes* is a name. The disease, diabetes, is a concept or idea that we form about a group of people who are similar with respect to difficulties in modulating their blood sugars. It is not a thing or a creature such as a rock, a bird, a building or a tree that has a discrete physical existence that is subject to individual observation and classification. In the 19th century natural scientists made huge strides in understanding the workings of the natural world by observing and then arranging or classifying living things as well as natural elements. The triumph of the natural order of biology and its classification led to an expectation that doctors could discover and classify all of the diseases and thereby gain a complete understanding of the nature of illness. Moreover, the discovery and identification of many germs as the cause of most acute illness gave realistic credence to the notion that actual entities were involved. In addition, most illnesses at the time were acute illnesses, so the distinction between the germ as a thing and the disease as an idea was, in a sense, academic.

We regularly hear at Grand Rounds and CPCs, as well as in the newspaper, that certain disease "entities" cause certain symptoms. Giving a disease a name is not the problem. Identifying the patient's problem, even if only by naming it, rescues the patient from the lonely fear that "no one knows what I have." The informal habit of referring to depression as the cause of sadness, colitis as the cause of diarrhea or arthritis as the cause of joint pain is not a bad one unless the speaker really believes that naming the problem is as helpful as finding the cause. The real value of giving a name to a problem is the same as the real value of the physician's first task: to do everything possible to rule out the really bad things that can happen to people.

When a child is told that dyslexia is the cause of his reading problem there is reason to be relieved that it is not from some less manageable cause. On the other hand, if the child could read he might understand that dyslexia is just a Greek word that means difficulty reading. If you believe that this is just a question of semantics, then consider the child who is hyperactive and cannot pay attention. If he or she is taken to a consultant who pronounces that the cause is attention deficit disorder with hyperactivity with the International Classification of Diseases code 314.01, it is easy to get the impression that the child is the victim of an attack from a disease entity. Then thinking can stop and prescribing can start. One does not have to ask questions as to whether this particular child has special unmet biochemical need or needs to avoid something to which he or she is sensitive. One can target the disease with the "treatment of choice" and give the child the group treatment, in this case a drug. It is not so much the drug that I am opposed to as it is the way of thinking. Nor do I want to do away with the names we use to describe illnesses. I want to do away with the implication carried by the names that distracts us from the very realistic possibility that a particular patient has detectable imbalances that constitute a cause or significant contributing factor to his or her problem.

The disease entity that has me most riled up lately is GERD. I see television ads in which a physician comes on to discuss heartburn and related symptoms. If you have these symptoms, says the doctor, you may have GERD, which stands for gastro-esophageal reflux disease. The name is quite descriptive of the probable mechanism of heartburn. It is certainly better than the word heartburn, which suggests a cardiac inferno. If they want to change the name of heartburn to GERD, I'm all for it. What exasperates me, however, is that the intent of the ad is to dignify the symptom as an entity, to cast the sufferer as a victim and to promote a drug that quenches stomach acid as the rescuer. The ad does not say "If you have GERD you may have a food allergy, a *Helicobacter pylori* or thrush infection and you should go to have these factors checked out." The ad shows how naming a problem, however inane the name might be, encourages the idea that "we know what you've got and here is what you should take for it."

If you get the idea that I am sour about the way drugs are used in our culture, you are right. In medical school I was taught that real doctors prescribe drugs and that any other approaches to illness except surgery and maybe psychotherapy, are invalid. The whole mentality about what constitutes a "scientific study" is engendered by drug trials in which two groups of people are treated for the same problem, but one group gets a drug and the other gets a placebo. There is no denying the validity of such an approach. It is, however, not the be-all-and-end-all of science. Biologists, physicists, chemists and engineers manage to observe nature and make discoveries without limiting themselves to double-blind placebo-controlled studies. Crookshank provides the two keys to the medical profession's capacity to participate in science with the same tools as other scientists. One is a general theory about how people get sick and the other is a language that reflects the reality of the subject. The theory, if you can call it that, that has dominated medical science for 70 years is that people get sick because they are the victims of disease entities. A *better theory,* in my opinion, is that people get sick because of a disruption of the dynamic balance that exists between themselves and their environment. That theory works just as well to describe what happens when you get chicken pox as it does when you have a more complex problem in which many genetic, environmental and nutritional factors interact. The medical language that was in place 70 years ago is the same as it is now: disease-oriented. If I am asked to name Seth's disease, I come up far short of really describing it. A *better language* is one in which all the details of a person's problems are preserved so that their individuality can be preserved.

The technology of computers can preserve a patient's individuality. We can make portraits of our patients' symptoms (what the patient reports), signs (what the doctor observes) and laboratory report results in a way that preserves individuality while keeping the names we use to describe the main features of illnesses. If we do that we have tools for observing nature in ways not previously available. Those ways depend on the capacity of computers to make pictures out of data. If the data is detailed, accurate and structured, the pictures will reflect reality and allow us to see patterns that are not visible to the naked eye. The computer can be a kind of macroscope for seeing large patterns just as the microscope is an instrument for seeing things that are infinitesimally small.

All that is needed is to put signs, symptoms and laboratory tests into a format that computers can use. Without a format that preserves the meaning of the language we use to describe signs, symptoms and lab tests, we end up with a chaos caused by synonyms. For example if a patient tells me he or she is sad, has a headache, or a pain in the abdomen, I may choose among many different words to express or record these problems. If the meaning of the words are transformed by giving them dimension, we enrich the words or language we use. We don't need to stop using the words, we just need a better way of keeping track of them, using a tool that will ultimately help us preserve the individual portrait of a problem more effectively than simply giving it a name.

Let me give you an example of what I mean by transforming the meaning of a word as applied to words describing symptoms. Symptoms take place in the human body where we have a common understanding of certain locations (head, chest, foot) where things can happen, certain body systems (skin, digestive, respiratory) that are involved and certain kinds of happenings or functions (pain, itching, increase or decrease in function) that describe the sensations or changes that we all experience when our bodies send us the messages we call symptoms. My job as a physician is to help my patients understand the meaning of various symptoms. Part of this job is the making of a record of the words my patients use to describe how they feel. It is easy enough to write down headache, itchy palms, or depression and then add detail as to when the symptom started, how long episodes last, how frequently the problem recurs, how severe it is, and how it is affected by various aggravating and alleviating factors. Using a computer it is also easy enough to record such symptoms so that the meaning of the word used to describe the symptom is transformed into a format that specifies the symptom's location, system and function.

Some years ago I began doing this on lined paper as I took histories from my patients. It was soon evident that a relatively small number of specific locations, systems and functions could be combined to give the meaning of a very large number of symptoms whose meaning would continue to reside in the words used by patients as well as in a more formal designation of the symptoms' "dimensions," their locations, systems and functions.

Here is how I would transform itchy palms, headache and depression into three dimensions describing location, system and function. Itchy skin is easy. The two words embody two dimensions, reassuring us that this new way of recording the meaning of what we are saying is not very different from our natural way of speaking.

The third dimension, skin, is implied when we say itchy palms, but when I transform the meaning from itchy palms to palms-skin-itching the implied part becomes explicit. Making it explicit is important because it may be helpful to be able to retrieve from the computer all of the information relative to skin.

Headache gets a little more complicated, but the two syllables of the word are easily mapped into two dimensions that can be put into rows and columns: the location—head and the function—pain. Headache has no system because the word *headache* does not convey any information as to whether it is related to the nervous system, the respiratory system (sinuses) or the muscular system (tension headache). Depression has to do with the system emotion. It has no location as such and its function is "decreased" because it is a symptom that represents a lowering of one's emotional state. The functional dimension of anxiety is "increased."

The portrait of a person complaining of itchy skin, headache and depression would look like this if we included only those features. This is not the sort of portrait that would be useful, but is only a cartoon to show you the principles involved in getting the words we use to describe symptoms into dimensions, which then can be put into rows and columns in a computer where their position preserves the meaning of the original symptom.

|  | Itching | Pain | Decrease |
|---|---|---|---|
| Skin | Itchy skin |  |  |
| Emotion |  |  | Depression |
| No system |  | Headache |  |

If we were to add several other functions, several more systems and all the places in the body we would be able to have a framework for preserving the individuality of the symptom pattern. If we added all laboratory results, also portrayed in rows and columns, the picture would become not only a way of making the portrait but of visualizing the ways it does or does not resemble others.

I have used such a system to record the symptoms of my pa-

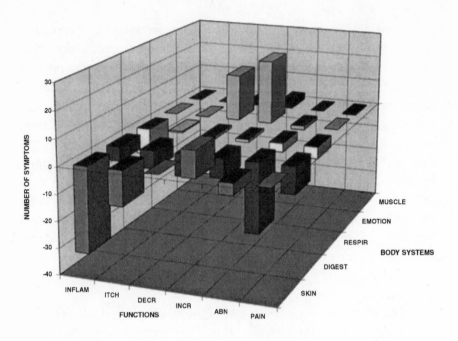

FIGURE 1

**Using the Computer to See Invisible Patterns in Groups of Patients**

tients and then made a picture using the computer to yield patterns that I could not see with the naked eye. I wanted to see the differences between two groups of patients whom I knew differed with respect to the results of a test for magnesium deficiency. One group had a normal test and the other group had an unusual result that no one knew how to interpret. When given magnesium by injection the second group "wasted" it by excreting all that was given plus a substantial amount more. This way of handing magnesium does not make sense. The test was performed to see if a patient retains a lot of the magnesium, which indicates that his body was deficient to begin with; if the magnesium is released, the body is saying, "Thanks, but I don't need it." I was puzzled by the magnesium wasters and I would have had no way of understanding this phenomenon if I had only a diagnosis to go by. My computer picture of the two groups could be manipulated to show the number of symptoms in the normal magnesium test group as compared with the magnesium wasters. Figure 1 shows how it looked when I subtracted the symptoms in the normal group from the symptoms in the waster group. The figure shows a version of the results that has been simplified by reducing the number of functions and systems shown. The bars that project below the plane of the diagram indicate symptoms that are less frequent in the wasters than in the patients with normal magnesium excretion. The bars that project above the plane show symptoms that are more frequent. Right away you can see that the magnesium wasters are individuals with significantly more emotional symptoms, such as anxiety and depression, and far fewer symptoms related to the skin and the digestive tract. Making this picture allowed me to see that the magnesium wasting group was real—not a statistical fluke or collection of laboratory errors. Being able to see the reality of the situation was the first step in understanding its meaning and knowing how to look for individuals with an unusual form of magnesium deficiency.

This technology applies the concepts of cyberhealth not only to individuals, but also to groups of patients, while avoiding the use of diagnostic labels. The more it appears that two individuals can "have the same thing," such as depression, colitis or arthritis from very different webs of interacting causes, the more important it is to be able to describe people in greater detail and individuality than is conveyed by diagnostic terms. Until the advent of computers, we did not have tools that could take us beyond the diagnostic labels we use to describe patients. Until the last 70 years, when complex chronic illness has become more common than simple acute illness in medical practice, we did not have such a great need for penetrating the complexity of illness with tools for seeing its invisibly large patterns. The map in chapter 14 is a guide for thoroughness that helps me answer the question Dr. Miller asked me when I worked with him in Kathmandu, "Sidney, have we done everything we can for this patient?" If I can also maintain and use a portrait of my patients' problems that is more detailed and accurate and structured than an old-fashioned diagnostic label, I will be living up to the maxims of Dr. Crookshank as well as Dr. Miller.

The outlook expressed in the previous few paragraphs looks farther to the future than the rest of the book, which describes a way of thinking about health and disease that is accessible to you now. It goes beyond the notion of making a diagnosis to considering the interaction between your body and its environment as well as the interactions between the many functions within your body. It does not pinpoint one body system to blame for your troubles. To the extent that this way of thinking is a guide to analyzing your problems it is a cybernetic approach to analysis. Maybe we could call it not psychoanalysis but ecoanalysis because it is fundamentally an ecological concept. If you take such an approach to health and illness you should know that it comes with a different kind of commitment—a commitment to change as compared with the old model—taking a pill to suppress a symptom.

Cyberhealth is based on the premise that illness is the result of a complex interaction of many factors that establish balance in the body. Even when a particular factor is known to cause a chronic illness, treatment should not stop at addressing that factor but should extend to all reasonable ways of establishing balance within the patient. The examples I have given in this book may give the paradoxical impression that there is usually a simple explanation for a person's problem and that the map is meant as a guide to finding that one cause.

I have used examples of illnesses with single causes to clarify the various possibilities that enrich the diagnostic process. Most of the time chronic illness has more than one contributing factor. The most important thing I have learned from being a doctor is that people who become sick in complicated ways, including people who become sick with potentially enduring or mortal problems, do best when they are able to change. I have participated in many discussions in which the question of "compliance" is raised by physicians who are skeptical of the role of diet, nutrition, exercise, meditation and other aspects of what has become known as lifestyle. "When people are sick," they say, "they have a hard enough time taking their medicine. All those other things just use up their energies so that they are, if anything, less likely to be compliant with appropriate medical treatments." It may be true that the "average person" just wants to take a pill and not be bothered by making changes. If so, this book is not for that person, unless it has not yet occurred to him or her that change is a possibility to consider.

The changes I have in mind differ from person to person. For some it means a new job, for others a new spiritual orientation and for others a change in their relationships with others. For many it means a change in their biochemistry, the subject I have addressed in this book. Those who can face choices without ambivalence do better than others. Those who do best are the ones who realize that they have been sitting on a need to change something and who understand the basic message of this book: illness is a signal to change.

# References

1. Smithells, R.W., Sheppard S., Schorah C.J. Vitamin deficiencies and neural tube defects. *Arch Dis Child* 1976 Dec;51(12):944–50.
2. Butterworth C.E. Jr. Folate status, women's health, pregnancy outcome, and cancer. *J Am Coll Nutr* 1993 Aug;12(4):438–41.
3. Shonenshine, D. Tick paralysis and other tick-borne toxicoses, in *The Biology of Ticks*, Vol II Oxford University Press. New York 1993.
4. Campbell, D.G. The ordeal of poor old charlie, "drunkless drunk." Los Angeles Times News Service, January 1983.
5. Crook, W. *The Yeast Connection*, Jackson TN: Professional Books, 1986.
6. Truss, O. *The Missing Diagnosis*. PO Box 26508, Birmingham, Alabama, 1982.
7. Coulter, H.L., *Divided Legacy*, 2nd ed, Richmond, CA: North Atlantic Books, 1982.
8. Weiss, Bernard. Food additives and environmental chemicals as sources of childhood behavior disorders, *Journal of the American Academy of Child Psychiatry*, 21, 2:144–152, 1982.
9. Donald Rudin, M.D. and David Horrobin, M.D. spent the weekend with a small discussion group of practitioners from the Northeast. With the help of two of our members, Leo Galland, M.D. and Neil Orenstein, Ph.D. we brainstormed the chemistry of fatty acids and prostaglandin hormones for three straight days. Few other educational experiences have so improved my ability to help my patients. Dr. Rudin's book, *The Omega Factor*, became the first of several references that elucidate the fatty acid problem. Dr. Galland's book *Superimmunity for Kids* (Dutton, 1988) is another excellent reference.

*Fats that Heal Fats that Kill* by Udo Erasmus (Vancouver, BC: Alive Books, 1993) also gives an excellent review of the subject.

10. Metametrix Laboratory, 5000 Peachtree Industrial Boulevard, Norcross, GA 30011. Tel.: 1-800-221-4640.

11. Siguel, E. M.D., Ph.D. P.O. Box 5, Brookline, MA 02146–0001, E-mail: nutrek@efafood.com, Home Page: www.efafood.com.

12. Siguel, E. *Essential Fatty Acids in Health and Disease.* 1994. Nutrek Press, P.O. Box 1269, Brookline, MA 02146.

13. Siguel, E., Lerman, R.H. Fatty acid patterns in patients with angiographically documented coronary artery disease. *Metabolism,* 1994: 43:982–993.

14. ———. Fatty acid patterns in patients with chronic intestinal disease. *Metabolism.* 1996; 45(1):12–23.

15. ———. The role of essential fatty acids: dangers in the USDA dietary recommendations ("pyramid") and in low-fat diets. *Am J Clin Nut,* 1994; 60:973–9 and *Am J Clin Nutr,* 1995; 63:973–9.

16. Siguel, E. Dietary sources of long-chain n-3 polyunsaturated fatty acids. *JAMA,* 1996; 275:836.

17. Siguel, E., Lerman R.H. The effects of low-fat diet on lipid levels. *JAMA,* 1996; 275:759.

18. Siguel E., Lerman R.H., MacBeath, B. Low-fat diets for coronary heart disease: perhaps, but which one? *JAMA,* 1996:275: 1402–1403.

19. Smigel, K. Beta carotene fails to prevent cancer in two major studies, CARET intervention stopped. *J Natl Cancer Inst,* 1996.

20. Baker, S.M. *Folic Acid.* Keats Publishing, Inc., 1995.

21. McCully, K.S. Vascular pathology of homocysteinuria: implications for the pathogenesis of arteriosclerosis. *Am J Pathol* 1969; 56:111–128.

22. Stamler, J.S., Slivka, A. Biological chemistry of thiols in the vasculature and in vascular-related disease, *Nutrition Reviews,* 1996;54:1, 1–30.

23. Clarke R., Daly L., Robinson K., et al. Hyperhomocysteine: an independent factor for vascular disease. *N Eng J Med* 1991;324:1149–55.

24. Baker, S.M. *Folic Acid,* Keats Publishing, Inc., 1995.

25. Rimland, Bernard, *Infantile Autism,* Englewood, NJ: Prentice Hall, 1964.

26. Dohan F.C. Cereals and schizophrenia—data and hypothesis. *Acta Psychiatr Scand* 1966;42:125.

27. Dohan F.C. Schizophrenia: possible relationship to cereal grains and

celiac disease. In S. Sankar (ed.) *Schizophrenia: Current Concepts and Research.* Hicksville, NY: P.J.D. Publications, Ltd., 1969:539.

28. Dohan, F.C. The possible pathogenic effect of cereal grains in schizophrenia—celiac disease as a model. *Acta Neurol.* 1976;31:195.

29. Dohan, F.C., Grasberger J., Lowell F., Johnston, H. Jr., Arbegast, A. Relapsed schizophrenics: more rapid improvement on a milk- and cereal-free diet. *Br. J. Psychiatry.* 1969;115:595.

30. Kinivsberg, A. M., Wiig K., Lind G., Nodland M., Reichelt K. L. Dietary intervention in autistic syndromes. *Brain Dysfunction,* 1990, 3, 315–327.

31. Reichelt, K. L., Ekrem J., Scot H. Gluten, milk proteins and autism: dietary intervention effects on behavior and peptide secretion. *Journal of Applied Nutrition,* 1990, 42(1):1–11.

32. Reichelt, K. L., Hole K., Hamberger A., Saelid G., Edminson P. D., Braestrup C. B., Lingjaerde O., Ledaal P. and Orbeck H. Biologically active peptide-containing fractions in schizophrenia and childhood autism. *Adv Biochem Psychopharmacol,* 1981, 28:627–43.

33. Reichelt, K. L., Knivsberg A. M., Lind G., Nodland M. Probable Etiology and Possible Treatment of Childhood Autism. *Brain Dysfunction,* 1991, 4:308–19.

34. Reichelt, K. L., Knivsberg A. M., Nodland, M., Lind, G. Nature and consequences of hyperpeptiduria and bovine casomorphins found in autistic syndromes. *Developmental Brain Dysfunction,* 1994;7:71–85.

35. Reichelt, K. L., Saelid G., Lindback T., Boler J. B. Child autism: a complex disorder. *Biological Psychiatry,* 1986, 21:1279–90.

36. Reichelt, K. L., Sagedal, E., Landmark J., Sangvik, B. T., Eggen, O., Scott, H. The effect of gluten-free diet on urinary peptide excretion and clinical state in schizophrenia. *Journal of Orthomoecular Medicine,* 1990, 5(4):223–39.

37. Shattock, P., Kennedy, A., Rowell, F., Berney, T. Role of neuropeptides in autism and their relationships with classical neurotransmitters. *Brain Dysfunction,* 1990, 3:328–345.

38. Williams, K., Shattock, P., Berney, T. Proteins, peptides and autism: part 1: urinary protein patterns in autism as revealed by sodium dodecyl sulphate-polyacrylamide gel electrophoresis and silver staining. *Brain Dysfunction,* 1991, 4:320–322.

39. Shattock, P., Lowdon, G. Proteins, peptides and autism: part 2: implications for the education and care of people with autism. *Brain Dysfunction,* 1991, 4:323–334.

40. Trygstad, O. E., Reichelt K. L., et al. Patterns of peptides and protein-

associated-peptide complexes in psychiatric disorders. *British Journal of Psychiatry*, 1980, 136:59–72.

41. *Additional peptide references:*

Asperger, H. Der psychopathologie des coeliakikranekn kindes. *Annal der paediatri*, 1961, 187: 346–351.

Axelsson, I. et al. Bovine beta-lactogobulin in human milk. *Acta Paed Scand*, 1986, 75: 702–707.

Bethou, J. et al. Immunostimulating properties and three-dimensional structure of two tripeptides from human and cow caseins. *Febs Letters*, 1987, 218:55–58.

Cornell, H.J. Amino acid composition of peptides remaining after in vitro digestion of a gliadin sub-fraction with duodenal mucosa from patients with coeliac disease. *Clin Chim Acta*, 1988, 176: 279–290.

DeGandiaras J.M. et al. Effects of acute lithium administration on pyrolgutamyl-aminopeptidase-1 activity in several brain areas of the rat. *Artzneimittel Forsch*, 1994, 44:119–121.

Gardner, M.L.G. Absorption of intact proteins and peptides. In Physiology of the gastrointestinal tract, ed. by L.R. Johnson, 3rd ed., Raven Press, 1994, 1795–1820.

Gillberg, C. et al. Endorphin activity in childhood psychosis. *Arch gen psychiat*, 1985, 42: 780–783.

Gobbi, G. et al. Coeliac disease, epilepsy and cerebral calcifications. *The Lancet*, 1992, 340:439–443.

Hallert, C. et al. Psychic disturbance in adult coeliac disease III. Reduced central monoamine metabolism and signs of depression. *Scand J Gastroenterol*, 1982, 17:25–28.

Husby, S. et al. Passage of undegraded antigen into the blood of healthy adults. *Scand J Immunol*, 1985, 22:83–92.

Israngkun P.P. et al. Potential biochemical markers for infantile autism. *Neurochem pathol*, 1986, 5:51–70.

Kahn, A. et al. Difficulty in initiating and maintaining sleep associated with cow's milk allergy in infants. *Sleep*, 1987, 10:115–121.

Kahn, A. et al. Insomnia and cow's milk allergy in infants. *Pediatrics*, 1985, 76:880–884.

Kinney, H.C. et al. Degeneration of the central nervous system associated with coeliac disease. *J neurol Sci*, 1982, 5: 9–22.

Klosse, J.A. et al. An automated chromatographic system for the continued analysis of urinary peptides and amino acids. *Clin Chim Acta*, 1972, 42: 409–422.

Knivsberg, A. M. et al. Dietary intervention in autistic syndromes. *Brain Dysfunct*, 1990, 3:315–327.

———. Autistic syndromes and diet: a four-year follow-up study of 15 subjects. *Scand J Educational Res.*: In press,

Koning, P.A.N. et al. Chronic haloperidol and chloropromazine treatment alters in vitro beta-endorphin metabolism in rat brain. *Eur J Pharmacol*, 1990, 97:15–20.

Konkoy, C.S. et al. Chronic treatment with neuroleptics alters neutral endopeptidase 24.11 activity in rat brain regions. *Peptides*, 1993, 14:1017–1020.

LeBoyer, M. et al. Difference between plasma N- and C-terminally directed beta-endorphin immunoreactivity in infantile autism. *Am J Psychiat*, 1994, 151:1797–1801.

Mahe, S. et al. Absorption of intact morphiceptin by diisopropyl-fluorophosphate-treated rabbit ileum. *Peptides*, 1989, 10: 45–52.

Migliore-Samour, D. and Jollet P. Casein, a prohormone with immunostimulating role in the newborns? *Experientia*, 1988, 44:88–93.

Murch et al. Disruption of sulphated glycosaminoglycans in intestinal inflammation. *The Lancet*, 1993, 341:711–714.

Paul, K.D. et al. EEG-Befunde bei zoeliakranken kindern in abh{ngigheit der ern{hrung. *Z Kilin Med*, 1985, 40:707–709.

Payan, D.G. et al. Specific high-affinity binding sites for synthetic gliadin heptapeptide of human peripheral blood lymphocytes. *Life Sci*, 1987, 40:1229–1236.

Reichelt, K.L. et al. Gluten, milk proteins and autism: results of dietary intervention on behavior and urinary peptide secretion. *J Applied Nutrition*, 1990, 42:1–11.

———. Nature and consequences of hyperpeptiduria and bovine casomorphins found in autistic syndromes. *Develop Brain Dysfunct*, 1994, 7:71–85.

———. Probable etiology and possible treatment of childhood autism. *Brain Dysfunct*, 1991, 4:308–319.

Reichelt, K.L. and Landmark, J. Specific IgA antibody increases in Schizophrenia. *Biol psychiat*, 1994, 37:410–413.

Reichelt, K.L. et al. Childhood autism: a complex disorder. *Biol psychiat*, 1986, 21:1279–1290.

Rostami, A. et al. Induction of severe experimental autoimmune neuritis with a synthetic peptide corresponding to the 53–78 amino acid sequence of the myelin P2 protein. *J neuroimmunol*, 1990, 30:145–151.

Shattock, P. et al. Role of neuropeptides in autism and their relationships with classical neurotransmitters. *Brain Dysfunct,* 1990, 3:328–346.

Stuart, C.A. et al. Passage of cow's milk protein in human milk. *Clin Allergy,* 1984, 14: 533–535.

Traficante, L.S. and Turnbull, B. Neuropeptide degrading enzyme(s) in plasma and brain: effect of in vivo neuroleptic administration. *Pharmacol Res Comm,* 1982, 14: 533–535.

Troncone, R. et al. Passage of gliadin into human breast milk. *Acta Paed scand,* 1987, 76: 453–456.

Werner, G.H. Natural and synthetic peptides (other than neuropeptides) endowed with immunomodulating activities. *Immunol Letters,* 1987, 16:363–370.

Wieser, H. Coeliac activity of the gliadin peptides CT-1 and CT-2. *Zeitschr Lebensmitteluntersuch Forsch,* 1986, 182: 115–117.

Wieser, H. et al. Amino acid sequence of the coeliac active gliadin peptide B 3142. *Zeitschr Lebensmitteluntersuch Forsh,* 1984, 79:3371–3376.

Zagon, I.S. and Mclaughlin, P.J. Endogenous opioid systems regulate cell proliferation in the developing rat brain. *Brain Res,* 1987, 412: 68–72.

42. Scriver, C.R. and Rosenberg, L.E. *Amino Acid Metabolism and its Disorders.* W.B. Saunders, 1973, p. 475.

43. Shaw, W., Kassen, E., Chaves, E. Increased urinary excretion of analogs of Krebs cycle metabolites and arabinose in two brothers with autistic features, *Clin Chem,* 1995, 41/8, 1094–1104.

44. Shaw, W., Chaves, E., Luxem, M. Abnormal urine organic acids associated with fungal metabolism in urine samples of children with autism: preliminary results of a clinical trial with antifungal drugs, *Proc of the National Autism Society of America,* July 1995.

45. Werbach, M.R., *Nutritional Influences on Illness.* Keats Publishing, Inc., 1988.

46. Adlercreutz, H. Lignans and isoflavonoids and their possible role in prevention of cancer. Paper presented at The Third International Symposium on Functional Medicine, Vancouver British Colombia, March 1996.

47. Greco, L., From the neolithic revolution to the gluten intolerance: benefits and problems associated to the cultivation of wheat. Internet posting on Cel-pro discussion group. June 30, 1995.

48. Greco L., Maki, M., Di Donato, F., Visakorpi, J.K. Epidemiology of

coeliac disease in europe and the mediterranean area. A summary report on the Multicentric Study by the European Society of Paediatric Gastroenterology and Nutrition. In *Common Food Intolerances 1: Epidemiology of Coeliac Disease,* Auricchio, S. and Visakorpi, J.K., editors. Karger, Basel, 1992, pp. 14–24.

49. Catassi C., Ratsch I.M., Fabiani E., Rossini M., Bordicchia F., Candela F., Coppa G.V., Giorgi P.L. Coeliac disease in the year 2000: exploring the iceberg. *Lancet,* 1994, 343: 200–203.

50. Kieffer, M., Frazier, P.J., Daniels, N.W.R. Coombs, R.R.A. Wheat gliadin fractions and other cereal antigens reactive with antibodies in the sera of coeliac patients. *Clin Exp Immunol,* 1982;50:651–660.

51. Finn, R., Harvey, M.M., Johnson, P.M., Verbov J.L., et al. Serum IgG antibodies to gliadin and other dietary antigens in adults with atopic eczema. *Clinical and Experimental Dermatology,* 1985;10:222–228.

52. Cohen, G., Hartman, G., Hamburger, R., O'Connor, R. Severe anemia and chronic bronchitis associated with a markedly elevated specific IgG to cow's milk protein. *Annals of Allergy* 1985;55:38–40.

53. Fallstrom, S.P., Ahlstedt, S., Carlsson, B., Lonnerdal, B., Hanson, A. Serum antibodies against native, processed and digested cow's milk proteins in children with cow's milk protein intolerance. *Clinical Allergy* 1986;16:417–423.

54. Shakib, F., Morrow Brown, H., Phelps, A., Redhead, R. Study of IgG sub-class antibodies in patients with milk intolerance. *Clinical Allergy* 1986;16:451–458.

55. Casimir, G.J.A. Duchateau, J., Gossart, B., Cuvelier, P.H. et al. Atopic dermatitis: role of food and house dust mite allergens. *Pediatrics* 1993;92:252–256.

56. Egger, J., Carter, C.M., Wilson, J. et al. Is migraine food allergy? A double-blind controlled trial of oligoantigenic diet treatment. *Lancet* 1983;ii:865–9.

57. Monro, J., Carini, C., Brostoff, J. Migraine is a food-allergic disease. *Lancet* 1984; ii:719–21.

58. Monro, J., Brostoff, J., Carini, C., Zilkha, K.J. Food allergy in migraine. *Lancet* 1980; ii:1–4.

59. Rowe, A.H. *Food Allergy: Its Manifestations, Diagnosis and Treatment.* Philadelphia: Lea and Febiger, 1931.

60. Rowe, A.H. Food allergy: its control by elimination diets. *Westminster Hosp Nurses' Rev* 1928; 13.

61. Shapiro, R.S., Eisenberg, B.C. Allergic headache. *Ann Allergy* 1965;23:123.

62. Grant, E.C.G. Food allergies and migraine. *Lancet* 1979;1:966.
63. Mansfield, L.E., Vaughan, T.R., Waller, S.F., Haverly, R.W., Ting, S. Food allergy and adult migraine: double-blind mediator confirmation of an allergic etiology. *Ann Allergy* 1985;55:126.
64. Williams, R. J. *Biochemical Individuality: the Basis for the Genetotrophic Concept.* New York: Wiley, 1956.
65. Stejskal, J.S., et al. Immunologic and brain MRI changes in patients with suspected metal intoxication. *Intl J Occup Med Toxicol,* 1995; 4: 1–9.
66. Stejskal, F.D.M. et al. MELISA, an *in vitro* tool for the study of metal allergy. *Toxic in vitro,* 1994; 8:991–1000.
67. Black, D.W., Ruthe, A., Goldstein, R.B. Environmental illness: a controlled study of 26 subjects with "20th century disease" *JAMA* 1990;264:3166–3170.
68. Ashford, N., Miller C. *Chemical Exposures: Low Levels, High Stakes.* New York: Van Nostrand, 1991.
69. Memorandum for All Regional Counsel from George L. Weidenfeller, Deputy General Counsel, U.S. Department of Housing and Urban Development, April 11, 1992, Subject: Multiple Chemical Sensitivity Disorder and Environmental Illness as Handicaps.
70. See: *Warmoth v. Bowen,* No. 85–2835 United States Court of Appeals, Seventh Circuit [798 F.2d 1109 (7th cir. 1986)] and *Kouril v. Bowen* No. 89–5187MN United States Court of Appeals, Eighth Circuit. [912 F.2nd 971 (8th Cir. 1990].
71. Rea, W., *Chemical Sensitivity,* Boca Raton: CRC Press.
72. Rogers, S., *Wellness At All Odds,* Syracuse, NY: Prestige Publishing, 1994. This is Dr. Rogers' most recent work and it cites her many other books and articles containing information and advice for patients.
73. Jefferies, W.M., *Safe Uses of Cortisone,* Springfield, IL: Charles C. Thomas, 1981.
74. Bower, L.P. Ecological chemistry. *Scientific American,* 1969;220;2, 22–29.
75. Husemann, Wolff, O., Husemann, F., *The Anthroposophical Approach to Medicine,* vol II. p 125. The Anthroposophical Press, 1987.
76. Tsalev, D.L., Zaprianov, Z.K. *Atomic Absorption Spectrometry in Occupational and Environmental Health Practice,* Boca Raton: CRC Press, Inc., p. 82, 1983.
77. Ganrot, P.O. Metabolism and possible health effects of aluminum. *Environ Health Persp,* 65: 363–371, 1986.

78. Galland, L., Barrie, S. *Intestinal Dysbiosis and the Causes of Disease.* Great Smokies Diagnostic Laboratory, Asheville, North Carolina, 1993.

79. Bland, J. Oxidants and antioxidants in clinical medicine: past, present and future. *J Nutr and Environ Med,* 1995:5;255–280.

80. Bland, J. *The 20-Day Rejuvenation Diet Program,* Keats Publishing, Inc. 1996.

81. Crook, W.G., *Tracking Down Hidden Food Allergies.* Jackson TN: Professional Books, 1990.

82. Bland J., Barrenger, E., Reedy R.G., Bland, K.A. A medical food-supplemented detoxification program in the management of chronic health problems. *Alternative Therapies,* 1995:1, 62–71.

83. Hildebrandt, G., Rhythmical functional order and man's emancipation from the time factor. In Schaefer, K.E., Hildebrandt, G., Macbeth, N., eds. *Basis of an Individual Physiology, A New Image of Man in Medicine Vol II,* New York: Futura Publishing Co., 1979, p. 19.

84. Samis, H. V. Jr., and Capobianco, S. Circadian dyschronism and chronotypic ecophilia as factors in aging and longevity. *Aging and Biological Rhythms,*1978 Plenum Publishing Corporation.

85. Ehret, C.D., Scanlon, L. *Overcoming Jet Lag.* Berkley Books, 1985.

86. Stough, C., Stough, R., *Dr. Breath, The Story of Breathing Coordination,* 1981, The Stough Institute, New York.

87. Crookshank, F.G. The importance of a theory of signs and a critique of language in the study of medicine, Supplement II in Ogden, C.K. and Richards, I.A. *The Meaning of Meaning,* New York: Harcourt Brace, 1923.

88. Brunjes, S. Yale clinical computer sciences project: development of a medical information science and its impact on health care systems and personnel, IBM Symposium 1970.

# Index

abnormalities, metabolic, 93–103
acetaminophen, 30, 146, 149, 160
acetate, 151
acid, 94
  organic, 98
acidophilus, 152
acne, 33, 35, 105, 134–135
acute, chronic compared to, 16, 21
addiction, 85
Adiercreutz, Herman, 106–107
adolescent, sexual development of, 23
adrenals, 24, 61
  insufficient, 132–136, 147
  stress and, 136
Africa, diets in, 104, 152
agent, etiologic, 20
AHTH, 82
airplane crashes, 28
AKG, 102, 140, 144
alcohol, 28
  negative effect of, 25, 41
  sensitivity to, 32
alcoholics, 25
Alka-Seltzer, 91
alkaline salts, 91
allergy, 41, 59,–51, 64, 125–127, 141
  avoidance of, 2, 25
  "sensitivity" and, 40
  testing for, 70
  respiratory, 37

alpha ketoglutarate (AKG), 102, 140, 144
alpha-linolenic acid, 61–63, 66
aluminum, 124, 143–144
amino acids, 51, 82, 88, 108, 140
  imbalance of, 131
  study of, 158
ammonia, 140, 152
ampicillin, 44, 46
anecdotal evidence, 48
anger, 70, 90, 136
animal dander, 124
antibiotics, 12, 33, 36, 86
antibodies, types of, 113
antihistamine, 91
antioxidants 65–84, 159
anxiety, 175–176
arthritis, 177
  food and, 44
  the word, 171
Ashford, Nicholas, 131
Asia, diets in, 104
asprin, 146, 149, 160
asthma, cat-induced, 42
attention deficit disorder, 171
autism, 26, 86–87, 90, 93, 157
Ayurvedic medicine, 168

B vitamins, 34, 83, 146
bacteria, and food, 52
Baker, Sidney, 190

baking soda, 91, 111
balance, xviii, 22, 98, 105, 128, 137, 173. See also Cyberhealth.
Barrie, Stephen, 155
benzoate, 147
beta-carotene, 70, 159
*bifidobacter*, 152
biochemestry, study of, 157
biologic toxins, 125
birth control pills, 12
birth defects, xv
Bland, Jeffrey, 157, 160
*blastocystis hominis*, 155
blood alcohol levels, 32
blood sugar levels, 99
blood, aluminum in, 144
*Borelia bergdorfi* germ, 21
bowel movements, 89, 99, 103
    of babies, 152
    rhythm of, 165
Bragdon, Henry, 160
brain waves, rhythm of, 163
breakfast, 166–167
breast buds, 23–26
breast cancer, 126
breathing
    diaphragmatic, 70
    rates, 162–165
Brunjes, Shannon, xvi, 170
Bueno, Herman, 155
Burkitt, Dennis, 104
butter, 59
butyrate, 151

cadmium, 82
caffeine, 146–148, 160, 166–167
CAH, 132–133
calcium, 122, 145–146
cancer chemotherapy, 36
cancer, 4, 64, 83, 102, 105
    breast, 105
    lung, 70
    prostate, 105, 108
Candida, 156
canola oil, 65
carbohydrates, 60–61, 166–167
carbon atoms, 29

carbon dioxide, 94, 152, 162, 168
cardiovascular disease, 80–81, 83
cats, allergy to, 41
Caveman Diet, 161
cedar, odor of, 126
celiac disease, 109–110
cells
    division of, 3
    permanent, 3, 6, 10–14
    transient, 4
cellulose, 108, 139
chemotherapy, 126
central nervous system, 1–9
champagne, 31
change, commitment to, 178–179
charcoal, 90
cheese, 40–41
chelation therapy, 146
chemical exposure, 129
chemicals, 124–125
chemistry screen, 12
"chicken skin," 54–55
child abuse, 136
chlorine, 143
cholesterol, 83
    stool tests and, 151
chromosomes, 73, 83
chronic, acute compared to, 16
chronology, personal, 126
ciliary action, rhythm of, 163
circadian rhythm, 164
citric acid, 95, 101, 144
clumsiness, motor, 54
cold sensations, 133–134
cold, 91
colitis, 177
    the word, 171
computers, cyberhealth and, 173–177
    individuality and, 173
concentrate, ability to, 4
conditioners, skin, 57, 66
congeners, 32
congenital adrenal hyperplasia (CAH), 132–133
Cook, Charles, 41
corn, cellulose fiber of, 150
coronary artery disease, 66

cortisol, 58
cortisone-like medicines, 133–134
cosmetics, 57, 66
cradle cap, 54, 57
Crook, William, 33, 35, 38, 161
Crookshank, F. G., 170, 177
cyberhealth, xv–xvi, xix, 158, 177–179
cyprohepatadine, 91
cysteine, 82
cytochrome P450, 142, 148

dander, 124–125
dandruff, 57
Davis, Adelle, 34
degradation, biologic process of, 25
dental cavities, 12
depression, 33–35, 175–176
  the word, 171
desensitization, 37
detoxification
  hormones and, 27
  markers, 150
  meaning of, xx
  testing, 139
  the word, 25
  the working of, 138–161
di-hydroxyphenylpropionic acid, 103
diabetes, the word, 171
diagnosis, xvi, 125
diagnostic labels, 170–179
diaper rash, 153
diaphragm, 167–168
diarrhea, 154, 171
diet, 178
  symptoms and, 35
  yeast-free, 37–38
digestion, 61
  disorders, 66
  problems, 93
  stool tests and, 149
digestive tract, surface area of, 151
disease entity, 170
disease, 21
  infectious, 38
  medicine and, 157
dissection, 6–7
diversity in insects, 122

dizziness, 134
DNA, 2, 83, 103–105, 144, 159
Dohan, F. C., 88–89
domino effect, 159
"Dr. Breath," 169
drugs, 22, 34, 83, 85, 137
  cancer, 102
  misuse of, 172
  trials, 172
dust, 124–125
Dwyer, John, 8
dysentery, 154
dyslexia, 171

E. coli, 152
ear wax, 18–19
earache, 44–46
ecoanalysis, 178
eczema, 33
eggs, 118–119
  allergy and, 41, 50–51, 64
empiricists, 37
encephalitis, 17
endorphins, 82, 86
enemas, 103
environment
  balance and, 173
  toxic, 82
enzymes, 29–30, 142
Epstein-Barr virus, 129
essential nutrients, 51
estrogen hormones, 23, 58, 80, 106
  detoxified, 41
  pesticides and, 27
Europe, diets in, 106
exercise, 58, 70, 178

fatigue, 34–35, 133–134
fats (lipids), 54–72, 159
  alcohol and, 29
  altered, 71
  hydrogenated, 71
  rancid, 52–53, 67–69, 71
  still, 71, 108
  stool tests and, 150
  trans, 71
fatty acids, 51, 57–59, 73, 125

rancid, 159
feet, painful, 54
Feingold, 46
fermentation, 28
feverfew, 82
fiber, dietary, 104–108
  stool tests and, 149
fingernails, brittle, 55–57
Finland
  diets in, 106, 111
  smokers in, 70
flavonoids, 159
flaxseed oil, 55, 65, 89, 108
flour, refined, 111
folic acid, xv, 77–78, 83, 105
food, 124–125
  baby, 152
  "drugs" in, 89
  additives, 47
  allergy, 44, 161
  cancer and, 107
  coloring, 45–47
  edibility of, 51
  GERD and, 172
  IgG class of, 113–116
  original not synthetic, 107
  peptides and, 75–92
  poisoning, 50–53
  preservative, 146
  rarity of, 44
  toxins and, 39–53
formula, baby, 152
free radicals, 76
functional medicine, 157
fungus, 100, 102, 154

Galland, Leo, 157
gamma strep, 152
gas, intestinal, 152
gastro-esophageal reflux disease
    (GERD), 172
genes, 73
genetic endowment, 73
genetics, mistakes and, 93–103
genitals, underdeveloped, 26
GERD, 172
germs, 125

aerobic, 152
Gesell Institute, 40
giardiasis, 154–155
globulins, 155–156
glucose, 28, 95, 101
glucuronic acid, 149
glucuronide, 142
glutamate, 140
glutamic acid, 82
glutamine, 140, 151
glutathione, 82, 102, 139, 146, 158–
    159
glycine, 82, 142, 144–145
glycogen, 58
gonads, 73
grains, 99
Greco, Luigi, 109–110
grief, 70
gut immunity, 155–157
gut, nutrition of the, 151

hair, 26, 64
  aluminum in, 144
  lead in, 146
  loss or growth, 57, 133–134
hangover, 91
hay fever, 42
headache, 39–42, 175. See also
    migraine.
Health Maintenance Organization, 42
health, problems with, 121–137
health-care system, xxi
heart disease, 64
heartbeat, rhythm of, 163
heartburn, 171
heavy metals, 25, 146
Helicobacter pylori, 93, 172
hepatitis, 53
hernia, 86
herpes simplex, 129
Hildebrandt, G., 164, 168
history, medicine and, 160
history, patient, 42–43
homocysteine, 78–84
  research in, 95
  testing for, 81–82
hormones, 58–61, 134

imbalance, 105
levels, 23–27
prostanoid, 58–59, 61, 64
"steroid," 58, 61
toxic, 23–27
host, susceptible, 20
hydrocortisone, 133–135, 157
hydrogenation, 64
hyperactivity, 47, 171
hypersensitivity, 127

IgG, 113–116
illness, 126
causes of, 173
roots of, 1–2
immune system, unity of the, 1–9
immunology, medicine and, 157
in vitro fertilization, 11
individuality, xxi, 20–22, 50, 122–134
computers and, 173
medicine and the, 157
patient's, 173
Pauling on, v
infection, 129
infertility, 10–14
inhalants, 124
intervention, 37
intestines, 151
leaks, 116–120
intolerance, 127
isoflavonoids, 106

jaundice, 86
Jefferies, William, 136
jet lag, 167
jobs, 126
joint paint, 44

kidneys, 140, 142
Krebs cycle, 95

lactic acid, 29
Lactobacillus, 108, 111, 152–153
lactulose, 116–118
lard, 59
lead, 82, 124
acetate, 145

paint, 145
poisoning, 146
Lebow, Avril, 20
Lee, Richard V., 6
lesion, cancerous, 55
Levin, Warren, 155
life events, invasive, 136
lifestyle, 178
light, 125, 166
lignans, 106
linoleic acid, 61–63
linseed oil. See flaxseed oil.
lipid peroxides, 159
lipids. See fats.
listening to patient, 44
liver, 25, 52, 58, 61, 141, 151
diaphragm and, 168
love, 125
low blood pressure, 134
lupus, 113
Lyme disease, 21
lymphocytes, 3

magnesium, 81, 128, 145, 157
magnesium deficiency, test for, 176
malaria, 16
malignancies, 83
mannitol, 116–118
margarine, 59, 64
Marshall, Barry, 93
Mayo-Smith, 61
McCully, Kilmer, 79–80, 93
McLellan, Bob, 126
MCS, 131
Mead acid, 66
meat, 27
estrogens and, 27
stool tests and, 149
medication, antifungal, 37–38
medicine, two camps in, v–vi, 157–159
meditation, 70, 178
Medrol, 133
"meeching look," 17
membranes
cell, 58
mucous, 58
memory, 4, 6, 8

Mendenhall, Thomas, 160
meningitis, 17
menstrual cycles, rhythm of, 164
mercury, 82, 122–125
metabolism
    antibiotics and, 99–101
    errors of, 97
metabolites, microbial, 98
Metchnikoff, Elie, 103
methionine, 78–79, 83, 143
methylation, 78
microbiology, 152
microorganisms, 124
"midnight ear," 17–18
migraine, 39, 113–119
    magnesium and, 157
    vitamin B6 and, 156
    See also headache,
milk
    breast, 142, 156
    cow's, 152
Miller, Claudia, 131, 177
Miller, Edgar, xvi-xviii
minerals, 125
    trace, 12–13, 34, 51
miso soup, 108
mold, 124–125
    food and, 37, 52
molecule
    carrier, 142
    degradation, 140
    making, 140
    synthesis, 140
morning sickness, 39
mucous membrane, 83
multiple chemical sensitivity (MCS),
    131
muscle weakness, 113
mycology, 154

nails, 64
naming an illness, 22
nausea, 39, 113
negative results, 45
nerve impulses, rhythm of, 163
nerve symptoms, peripheral, 35
nervous system, central, 4–6

neurological symptoms, 32
neurotransmitters, 101
nightshades, joint pain and, 44
nitric oxide, 160
nitrogen, 79
No-Doz, 146, 148
norepinephrine, 78
North American diet, 1543
numbness of hands and feet, 34
nutrition, 125, 178
nuts, 65
nystatin, 100

odor, intestinal function and, 153
Ogden, C.K., 170
oil
    rancid, 59–60, 67–69
    body 57, 66
    stiff or flexible, 55
olive oil, 59
omega–3 fatty acids, 55, 62–63, 66
one-sidedness, 113
operations, 126
opioid addiction, 91
opioids, 86
opium, 85–86
orange juice, 35
ovaries, 61
oxidation, 67–69
    stress and, 72–84, 159–161

paint, lead-based, 145
Pangborn, Jon, 157–158
Pap smear, 37
parasites, intestinal, 109–110, 154–155
parasitology, 13, 154
Parrish, Louis, 155
paste, 111
Pasteur, Louis, 30, 103
patient-centered diagnosis, 157
Pauling, Linus, v, 156
penicillin, reaction to, 44
penis, size of, 26
pentachlorophenol, cancer and, 126
peptides, 75–92
    endorphin-like, 90
perfumes, sensitivity to 87

peristalsis, rhythm of, 163
permeability testing, 116–120
peroxidation, 69
perspiration, 25
pesticides, estrogen and, 27
petrochemicals, 124–125
pH, 152
phenosulfotransferases (PST), 26
physical exam, 42–43
placebo, 172–173
poisons, 138
poisoning, food, 50–53
pollen, 124–125
pollutants, 82
potassium, 143
potassium bitartrate, 111
prednisone, 133–135
premenstrual syndrome, 91
propionate, 151
prostanoid hormones, 58–59, 61, 64, 66
prostate cancers, 108
PST, 26
protein, 60–61, 78, 88, 140, 155, 166–167
psychoanalysis, 178
psychotherapy, 172
ptomaine poisoning, 52
public policy, xxi

questionnaire, 126

radiation, 36
rage, 54
Randolph, Theron, 131
rash, 35
rationalists, 37
Rea, William, 132
reactive oxygen species, 76
recognition, 5–6
red dye, 46
Redlich, Fritz, xvi
reduced glutathione (RG), 69, 82
Reichelt, Karl, 87–89
Remington, Charles, 122
respiratory rate, 163
RG, 69, 82

rheumatic fever, 36
rhythm, 125, 152–169
Richards, I.A., 170
Rimland, Bernard, 87
Rogers, Sherry, 132
root of illness, 2
Rosenberg, Leon, 95–96, 156
Rubenstein, 157
rumen, 139
rye fiber, 106, 108–111

saccharine, 145
salad oil, 59
salicylic acid, 149
salt craving, 134–135
SAM, 74–84, 102
school performance, 54
schooling, 126
"scientific study," 172–173
Scriver, C.R., 96
seasonal cycles, rhythm of, 164
seborrhea, 57
sedatives, 141
seeds, 65
Seen, Milton, 40
Selye, Hans, 135–136
semantics, 171
senses, 4–6
sensitivity, 40
  to food, 109–120
  to smell and sound, 86
serotonin, 78
sesame seed, 108
sexual abuse, 136
shampoos, skin, 57
Shattock, Paul, 87
Shaw, William, 93–94, 98–103, 155
shock, anaphylactic, 41
Siguel, Eduardo, 66
singing, 167
sinuses, 175
skin, 64, 175
  alligator, 57
  dry, 55–57
sleep, rhythm of, 165
smell, sense of, 51, 67
smoking, tobacco, 70

sodium, 91, 143
sodium benzoate, 146, 148
sodium bicarbonate, 91, 111
somnolence, 113, 118
South America, diets in, 105
soy protein, 106–108
speech development, 86
steroids, 58, 61, 135
stomach acid, pH of, 152
stool analysis, 13, 116, 149–151
stool, pH of, 152
    alkaline, 152
    odor of, 153
    parasites and, 154–155
    tests of triglycerolides, 151
stress, 168
successes, 126
sugars, 28, 108, 142
    diet and, 12
sulfa drugs, 36
sulfate, 80
sulfur, 78, 143, 149
sunburn, 159
superoxide dismutase, 72
supplements, 84, 89, 98
    mineral, 34
    pharmaceuticals and, 84
    vitamins, 34, 70–72
    See also B vitamins and individual
        vitamins.
surgery, 172
suspension, pink, 46
sweetener, artificial, 145
symptoms, xvi
    chronic, 123
    "dimensions" of, 174–175
    patients', 173
    suppressing, 22
synthesis, biologic process of, 25
systems, the word, xvi
    theory of, xvii

taste of food, 51, 67
taurine, 78, 88
tea, 108
teeth, 12
testicles, 61

    size of, 26
testosterone, 58, 106
tetracycline, 33, 35
Three Mile Island, disaster at, 166
3-oxoglutaric acid, 102
thrush infection, 36
thyroid, 58, 61, 78
TIA, 113, 118–119
tick toxicosis, 19–21, 25, 41, 64
tingling in fingers and toes, 35
tobacco smoking, 70
tofu, 108
tonsillectomy, 136
toxins, 2, 15–22, 25, 28–38, 124–125,
        139, 146
    detoxification and, 27
    foods, 50–52
    hormones and, 27
    intestinal, 34
    testing for, 70
    yeast, 41
transient ischemic attack (TIA), 113,
        118–119
travelers, rhythms and, 167
"treatment of choice," 172
triglycerolides, 151
Truss, Orian, 36–38
tryptophan, 78
Tylenol, 146, 149
tyramine, 40–41
tyrosine, 78

ulcers, 105
    stomach, 93
UltraClear, 161
urine
    aluminum in, 144–145
    analysis, 160

vaginal infection, 36
valine, 95
vegetable oil, 59
verbalizing feelings, 70
virus, 16, 129
    hepatitis and, 53
vision, partial loss of, 39
visual symptoms, 113

vitamin B6, 79, 81, 83, 156
vitamin B12, 79, 81, 83, 96–97
vitamin C, 68–72, 75, 146, 159
vitamin E, 65–72, 82, 159
vitamins, 13, 51, 96, 125
    intolerance, 34
    supplements, 34
    See also individual vitamins.
vomiting, 39, 113

Warring, Rosemary, 26
waste, domestic, 82
water, 53
Weed, Lawrence, 43
Williams, Roger, 121, 123
wind instruments, playing, 167

wine-making, 30–31
withdrawal symptoms, 89
worms, 154
Wu, Nelson, xvi

x-rays, 75–77

yeasts, 30, 154
    avoidance of, 37
    baker's or brewer's, 35
    foods and, 35
    infection and, 21, 36, 129
    intestinal, 32–34
    problem, 155, 158
    reactions, 118

# About the Author

Sidney MacDonald Baker, M.D. is a practicing physician in Weston, Connecticut. His special interest is the environmental and biochemical aspects of chronic health problems of both children and adults. He is a graduate of Yale University and Yale Medical School and is board certified in obstetrics and pediatrics. Dr. Baker served in Chad, Africa as a Peace Corps volunteer, worked as a family practitioner in an H.M.O., was director of the Gesell Institute of Human Development and has taught at Yale Medical School and Southern Connecticut State University.

The author of dozens of popular and scientific articles about nutritional biochemistry and a popular lecturer on the subject, Dr. Baker is also the author of *Folic Acid* (Keats Publishing, Inc., 1995) and co-author, with Louise Bates Ames and Frances Ilg, of *Child Behavior* (Harper & Row, 1982) and *The Years from Ten to Fourteen* (Delacorte, 1988).